Pregnancy, Children & *the Hallelujah Diet*®

BY OLIN ID[...] C.N.C.

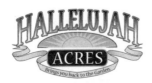

Authored by Olin Idol

Layout and Design by ⊕AdvanceGraphics (www.advancegraphics.us)

First printing 2002
Second printing 2005

ISBN 0-929619-12-9

This Edition Published and Distributed by

    Hallelujah Acres Publishing
    P.O. Box 2388
    Shelby, NC 28151
    704-481-1700

Visit our web site at http://www.hacres.com

Contents

ACKNOWLEDGEMENTS

I would like to express my deepest appreciation to all those who shared their testimonies with me concerning their experiences with a primarily raw plant–based diet and its impact on their pregnancy, delivery, and nourishment of their infants and children. I regret that limited space prohibits publishing each of these wonderful testimonies.

I would like to acknowledge the following wonderful ladies whose testimonies are dispersed throughout this book: Tina Fillmer, Carrie Malkmus, Doreen Martin, Susan Matchett, Stephanie McGovern, Nicole Nixon, Allie Olsen, and Kathy Raine. Thank you for your contributions, which illustrate the superiority of a primarily raw plant–based diet in meeting the nutritional needs of pregnancy and childbirth.

I am indebted to my wife, Myra, for the support and encouragement she has provided since I left a successful insurance career in 1995 and actively pursued a full–time career in health and nutrition, and went on to join Rev. George Malkmus and Hallelujah Acres®.

I would also like to express my appreciation to Rev. Malkmus for giving me the opportunity to minister to countless individuals as they pursue their goal of overcoming illness and achieving optimal health by adopting the Hallelujah Diet and Lifestyle.[SM]

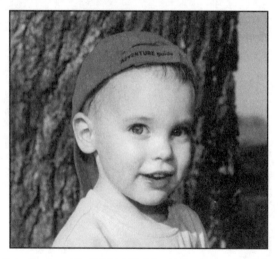

Parker Grassle—on The Hallelujah Diet® since birth and a strong healthy boy.
If it's not a raw fruit or vegetable he doesn't want it.

FOREWORD

By Rev. George H. Malkmus

When Olin Idol first joined our staff as my personal assistant here at Hallelujah Acres® in 1995, little did I realize the precious jewel God was sending our way! When Olin began, he handled most of my personal calls and correspondence. Because of his constant communication with people contacting him with questions, the answers to which he wasn't always sure, Olin started taking college courses in the subject of diet, nutrition, health, and related subjects to better qualify him to help these people. This resulted in his obtaining a Doctorate in Naturopathy, along with becoming a Certified Nutritional Consultant.

As time went by, Olin realized that almost everyone who applied The Hallelujah Diet® and the Biblical nutritional principles we were teaching, got well from whatever physical problem they were experiencing. Thus, The Hallelujah Diet® was found to be a tool for multitudes of people to regain and/or to maintain excellent health. We have received tens–of–thousands of testimonies from people who have experienced incredible healing after adopting The Hallelujah Diet®.

 It wasn't long before we learned that women were going through pregnancy on The Hallelujah Diet®, bearing children while on the diet, nursing these children while on the diet, and feeding these children based on the diet. This opened up a whole realm of new questions we hadn't dealt with before—questions that needed accurate answers. And so, once again, Olin came to the rescue and started researching the subject of pregnancy, children, and The Hallelujah Diet®.

There was very little information available on the subject of pregnancy, nursing, and raising children on a basically raw food diet. So, much of what Olin learned was based on the results mothers were experiencing on the diet. Our own Ph.D., Michael Donaldson, also started doing abundant research on the subject and sharing his findings with Olin.

This book, *Pregnancy, Children & the Hallelujah Diet®,* is the most comprehensive study of which I am aware on this subject. It shows the importance of vitamin B12 in the mother's diet during pregnancy and nursing, the vital role that proper fats play in the child's brain development, along with a multitude of other issues absolutely essential to delivering a healthy baby and to raising a healthy child.

I believe every parent, who desires to have a healthy baby and raise a healthy child, needs to read this book. But more than that, I believe every parent and grandparent should read this book. I know of no other place you can find this vital information.

I am personally thrilled that my daughter–in–law, Carrie Malkmus, followed the principles in this book to deliver two healthy Hallelujah babies. Both received an Apgar score of ten at birth. As of this writing, Zackary is six months old and thriving, while his brother Dylan is two and a half years old and already knows the alphabet, his colors, and can count to twenty. I fully endorse the information in this book, and I guarantee I want my grandchildren raised on its teachings.

Based on my 26 years of personal research and experience, Olin's seven years of research, listening to personal testimonies of what works and doesn't work, and the research of Michael Donaldson, Ph.D., I honestly believe you cannot find a better or more accurate source of information on pregnancy and child–raising than you will find in this book.

INTRODUCTION

And Adam knew Eve his wife; and she conceived, and bare
Cain, and said, I have gotten a man from the Lord.
—Genesis 4:1

Lo, children are an heritage of the Lord: and the
fruit of the womb is his reward.
—Psalm 127:3

From the very first conception and birth, God's plan for the pro-
creation of the human race has been fulfilled through the God–
given desire of a couple to marry, conceive, give birth, and rear
healthy, godly children who would then do likewise. Sadly, however, we
find ourselves living in an age when many couples have found themselves unable to experience the blessings of having children. We are
constantly exposed to innumerable environmental hazards and toxins
as well as mercury amalgam fillings in our teeth, dangerous childhood
vaccines, and nutritionally deficient food sources all resulting in a body
so overloaded with internal toxicity that it is unable to reproduce. John
Robbins (in a book first published in 1987) states, "Tests done at several
major universities have found that nearly 25% of today's college stu-
dents are sterile. This is a terrifying trend. Only thirty–five years ago,
the sterility rate was less than one–half of one percent."[1]

Testimony: Doreen Martin writes the following in a testimony
to Hallelujah Acres: *"I was not able to get pregnant for seven years*
after my first child. I was told about The Hallelujah Diet® and was
on it for fifteen months when I became pregnant and subsequently
miscarried. I continued on the diet and became pregnant again
two months later. I stayed faithfully on the dehydrated barley juice
powder throughout my pregnancy but no carrot juice. My doctor

was afraid of too much vitamin A during the first trimester. (I know now it would have been OK). I had a beautiful baby girl on January 19, 2000, and she has never been sick or had an ear infection and is a year old. I also did not vaccinate her after reading your book on vaccinations. . . . Your information has changed my life and my family's."

Note: Concerning vitamin A toxicity from *Understanding Nutrition,* "Beta–carotene, which is found in a wide variety of plant foods, is not converted efficiently enough in the body to cause a vitamin A toxicity; instead, it is stored in the fat deposits under the skin. Over–consumption of beta–carotene may turn the skin yellow, but this is not harmful. . . . A 1–cup serving of carrots, sweet potatoes, or dark greens such as spinach provides such liberal amounts of carotenoids that even allowing for inefficient absorption and conversion, the intake is sufficient for many days."[2]

How can a young couple that desires to have healthy children best prepare their bodies for the awesome responsibility of pregnancy? And, once a child has been born, how can they nourish that child for optimal development? If a couple already has children, how can they help transition these children to an optimal diet and lifestyle? These are some of the issues this book will address in an effort to help readers along their journey to ultimate health.

This book is written with the assumption that the reader is already familiar with the Hallelujah Diet & Lifestyle℠. For those of you who are not, please read a copy of *God's Way to Ultimate Health* by Rev. George H. Malkmus and a copy of *Recipes For Life . . . from God's Garden* by Rhonda Malkmus and begin educating yourselves as to the ideal way to nourish your bodies based on the concepts and natural laws established by God in Genesis 1:29. (See the back pages for order information.) We will not take the time to deal with the basics already established in these books, but will rather deal with some of the issues facing those concerned with preparations for and actually rearing children in accordance with the Hallelujah lifestyle. This information is not intended to be all–inclusive in regards to rearing and to feeding children, but seeks to address some of the varying needs of children on The Hallelujah Diet®. My objective is to offer general and practical guidelines for rearing healthy children on a primarily raw plant–based diet rather than offer a list of specifics. Each individual and family is different. I do not propose to offer a tailor–made lifestyle or diet that is to be followed to the letter, but rather offer fundamentals for consideration as you prepare to rear healthy children in accordance with God's natural laws.

It is the responsibility of each individual to educate himself on the basic concepts of optimal health and God's natural laws, and to learn how to properly care for the marvelous body temple with which God has blessed each of us. By doing our part, each of us can enjoy optimal health and have a body that functions in a manner compatible with God's plan for our lives. Throughout this book, you will read excerpts of testimonies from women who have experienced the challenges, as well as the rewards, of following The Hallelujah Diet®. I trust that God, through the ministry of the Holy Spirit, will open your mind and direct you in all truth as you read the following chapters. I pray that you will be stimulated and challenged to take responsibility for your own health, as well as that of your children.

> **Testimony:** Nicole Nixon from Texas shares the following with us: *"The biggest struggle has been breaking cravings/addictions and getting past mental issues with food. But the wonderful changes and results we have experienced have far outweighed any struggles we have had along the way. We are to the point now where we are 'in love' with our new way of eating and no longer feel 'deprived' because we cannot eat the foods that were ultimately killing us.*
>
> *"It was really tough for me, personally, to make a drastic diet change during the same time that my body was so drastically changing due to being pregnant. The cravings for killer foods were horrible. But it was so important to make this change at such a critical time. I wanted to create a healthy baby. I read* God's Way to Ultimate Health *and learned exactly how to eat in order to nourish my unborn child."*

CHAPTER 1

General Perspective on Nutrition Regarding Conception and Pregnancy

And God said, Behold, I have given you every herb bearing seed, which is upon the face of all the earth, and every tree, in the which is the fruit of a tree yielding seed; to you it shall be for meat.
—*Genesis 1:29*

In the Bible dictionary of the *Dickson New Analytical Study Edition of the King James Version Bible* under the definition of food we read, "The diet of the Hebrews in Palestine was almost entirely vegetarian. Meat was eaten occasionally by the rich."[3] It is interesting to see just how far we have departed from the Word of God today in questioning His ideal provisions for mankind.

One question that often looms in the mind of those preparing for conception is, "Can a healthy pregnancy be created and sustained, resulting in a healthy, full–sized, strong child on a diet devoid of meat and dairy products?" Fortunately, we are now seeing many of those in the traditional medical field recognize that not only is this possible, but also that it may very well be the optimal path to follow. One such noted authority in this area is Michael Klaper, M.D., author of *Pregnancy, Children, and the Vegan Diet*.[4]

Interestingly, in 1997 the American Dietetic Association's position paper on vegetarian diets stated, "Appropriately planned vegan and lacto-ovo-vegetarian diets satisfy the nutrient needs of infants, children, and adolescents and promote normal growth."[5] And in the seventh edition of *Dr. Spock's Baby and Child Care*, Dr Spock recommends a vegan diet for children.[6]

In his March/April 1997 newsletter, Dr. John McDougall relates his wife Mary's experience early on in their conversion to a strict vegetarian diet. Shortly after the birth of their second child in 1975, they had completed their transition to a strict vegetarian diet. He then states, "Five years later Mary became pregnant with our third. In no time she began buying cheese, fish, and eggs, reverting to old reasoning that this high-protein, high-calcium food was essential for a healthy pregnancy—even though I suspected she knew better. At three months, she had a miscarriage. This traumatic event caused her to rethink her decisions. Two years later, she was pregnant again. I waited for the return of cheese, or at least some fish, into our household—it never happened. Her experience of losing the last baby had cured her of fear-driven action. During the entire nine months of pregnancy, she had no meat, foul, fish, or dairy products—please note: not that these foods had necessarily caused her previous miscarriage, but that the introduction of these foods last time had not actually guaranteed a successful pregnancy."[7]

Mary McDougall reported she was very energetic every day, had no swelling, and gained only twenty pounds. After her son's birth, she was only five pounds heavier than her normal weight before pregnancy, and in a week, she lost the extra five pounds. She testifies that this was one of the healthiest and happy periods of her life.

It is amazing how many times we are driven to make decisions based on fear or peer influence rather than knowledge. Pregnancy is the time when a woman should be in optimal health. Unfortunately, for the vast majority of women, this is a time of being sick, overweight, constipated, and generally uncomfortable. Dr. McDougall states, "Many are on medications for diabetes and high blood pressure. For one-fourth of these pregnant women, the grand finale of this life-giving orchestration ends in surgical removal of the baby. Often at the source of all this trouble are doctors, dietitians, mothers, and mothers-in-law telling the mother-to-be to drink at least four glasses of milk a day for calcium and to eat plenty of meat for protein every day."[8]

It is important that mothers-to-be take the time and expend the effort to fully educate themselves in the area of optimal nutrition. The health and well-being of their children depends heavily upon the choices the mother will make in this area.

Learning From Natural Laws of Nature

When we look at nature, every animal creation of God (other than man) thrives and reproduces on a diet of all raw natural foods. This still holds true for every creature in the wild where man has not interfered, from the carnivore to the herbivore. Isn't it fascinating that an elephant can survive in the jungle and obtain all of the protein, calcium, and other nutrients necessary for reproduction of healthy offspring from a 100% raw plant-based diet? God in His wisdom made preparations in nature for all of His creation to be completely nourished, as we see in Genesis 1:29-30.

When God created Adam and Eve, he created them with a body capable of enjoying eternal life here on earth in a perfect environment in a physical body nourished exclusively with raw foods as served up by nature. I have no doubt that had Adam and Eve remained obedient to God and simply refrained from yielding to Satan's temptations, mankind could have enjoyed eternal life here on the earth in a body nourished perfectly with raw foods. Genesis 3:22-24 tells us that God drove Adam and Eve out of the Garden of Eden and placed cherubim and a flaming sword to guard the way to the tree of life lest they eat of it and live forever. It stands to reason that if God designed these bodies originally to be sustained on a raw plant-based diet, then that is the ideal way to nourish them today. Can man improve on God's provisions by processing and cooking his foods?

I realize that we no longer live in a perfect environment. Many changes have taken place since the original creation was destroyed by a flood some 1600 years after man first sinned. (We don't know how long Adam and Eve lived prior to sinning. Prior to sin, time was not an issue.) Yet, the basic concept of God's original diet for man can still be applied to us today, resulting in optimal health. As we adopt a primarily raw plant–based diet, it is important for us to take into consideration changes that have occurred in our food supply due to mankind's poor stewardship of God's natural resources. We will look more closely at these a little later when we look at specific nutritional needs.

Planning for Pregnancy

When a couple begins thinking in terms of a pregnancy, they must realize that it is vitally important that each of them nourish their body in the most optimal way possible. This should begin at least six months prior to the time of conception if at all possible. It is vital that the male's sperm and the female's egg be in the best condition possible before they are joined together. That single fertilized cell will, during the next approximately 270 days, grow and develop into a complex, organized human being ultimately consisting of nearly one hundred trillion cells. The initial quality of each individual cell will be dependant upon the nutrition that is provided through mother's diet. Life begins, is maintained, and ends at the cellular level. It is also important to realize that harmful substances, such as drugs, caffeine, and chemicals found in animal products, as well as the good nutrition, can pass through the placenta to the fetus. Thus, it is vitally important that the harmful substances be eliminated from the diet while optimal nutrition is provided.

We can easily see how critical good nutrition is from the outset. As noted by Virginia Messina and Mark Messina, it is vital that the father provide a healthy, well–nourished sperm to fertilize mother's equally healthy egg to give the baby the best start possible:

> "By the twentieth day after conception, the embryo is just one–tenth of an inch long and doesn't look even remotely like a baby, but it has a weakly beating heart and is beginning to develop eyes, a spinal cord, a nervous system, lungs, and intestines.

> "By the third week, the neural tube, which will become the brain and spinal cord, has formed. This is of great significance: failure of the neural tube to close properly can result in a host of common birth defects, including spina bifida. Researchers think that neural–tube defects may be the result of nutrient

deficiencies. A lack of the B vitamin folic acid is thought to lead to neural–tube defects.

"The fourth through the eighth weeks of pregnancy are the most critical in all human development. Drugs, alcohol, or extreme malnutrition can disturb the process of development at this point. By the end of eight weeks, the growing baby is no longer an embryo but is called a fetus, a Latin word meaning young one."[9]

Dr. Klaper adds: "The human body runs extremely efficiently on foods derived exclusively from plant sources, as basic textbooks in biochemistry or physiology will confirm. Creating a balanced, fully nutritious vegan diet is not difficult; however, a woman or couple choosing vegan nutrition for themselves and for their children must take seriously their responsibility for learning the fundamentals of what their bodies require, and what foods will meet those requirements."[10]

This is the underlying responsibility of any couple that is anticipating having a child. They certainly can't depend on the medical community to provide them with the nutritional knowledge required to rear healthy children. How many doctors do you know who are qualified to teach a person how to nutritionally care for their body?

Testimony: Nicole Nixon from Texas: *"When I was pregnant I had dehydrated barley juice powder and fresh carrot juice first thing in the morning. Then, the next time I felt hungry I would drink a big glass of water. Fresh fruit, usually two big apples and a banana, was what I needed mid–morning. Then at lunch, I would run all kinds of veggies through the juicer, switching from day to day to make sure I was getting every kind of nutrient from every kind of veggie. Carrots first, then I added to it celery, parsley, bell peppers, spinach, or beets, etc. I will be honest, the nausea thing was going on big time with me, and I had to hold my nose and guzzle my veggie juice, followed by a big swig of water to wash my mouth out before I could unplug my nose. For some reason, when I was pregnant, the smell and taste of the veggie juice was nauseating. Now that I'm not pregnant anymore, I can easily drink my juice, slowly, even swishing it around in my mouth before swallowing it, and I actually enjoy it.*

"I would wait 30 minutes after the juice, then have lunch. Some days I would make a big shake by blending together two frozen bananas, 1-cup fresh apple juice, and 1 cup frozen strawberries (or blueberries) for lunch. Other days, I would make a huge salad with lettuce, tomato, cucumber, avocado, olives, and my favorite salad dressing . . . A lot of the time, I had a big baked potato topped with olive oil . . . or a big bowl of pasta with my lunchtime salad. I also enjoyed an occasional veggie sandwich for lunch (whole grain bread such as Ezekiel from the health food store, spread with mashed avocado and topped with tomatoes and lettuce and sometimes cucumbers). In the afternoon I would get hungry again and first drink a huge glass of water, then eat soaked nuts (measure out nuts and cover with water, soak overnight, drain water and keep the nuts in a baggie in the refrigerator) or dried fruit or another couple of apples.

"Before supper I would make more veggie juice, then a salad or blended salad. The blended salads are great for when you know you need to eat a salad but don't feel like eating a salad. You just blend up all the veggies for your salad, get a big spoon so you can take big bites and get it over with; it's not very appetizing, but at least you're getting the good stuff in your body. Another favorite was to have raw soup instead of a salad (for when you start getting tired of salad all the time). Rhonda's book Recipes for Life has great raw soup recipes. Then we would have something cooked. To end the day, and because I was always hungry before bed, I would have another glass of fresh veggie juice or apple juice or another apple."

When we look around at most babies born of parents on the typical American diet, we find a host of nutritionally related problems, from re-occurring ear infections to colic and diaper rash. We see basically a whole generation of babies who are constantly in and out of the doctors' offices, on and off drugs continually. Is it any wonder we are seeing chronic disease in younger and younger children? We must shift our thinking away from the "medical mentality" that has been forced upon us for hundreds of years. The idea that the doctor is responsible for our health has resulted in a dismal failure. We can no longer continue as victims of the present day mindset, but must take responsibility for our own health as well as that of our children. The human body cannot be drugged into health. We must make that paradigm shift in our thinking if we are to enjoy optimal health.

Thousands of individuals have adopted the underlying concepts of The Hallelujah Diet® and have given remarkable testimonies of healings from such conditions as cancer, heart disease, diabetes, multiple sclerosis, and a host of other chronic degenerative conditions. Literally thousands more who were not experiencing any known physical problems have adopted The Hallelujah Diet® simply as a means of providing optimal nutrition and cleansing for the body so that they could attain and maintain optimal health. A number of couples who for various reasons were unable to get pregnant while eating the SAD (Standard American Diet) have found that within a few months of following The Hallelujah Diet® conception did occur, and ultimately they were able to deliver a strong healthy child.

Dr. Klaper stated the importance of nutrition well when he wrote: "It is clear that within minutes of eating anything, elements of that food are flowing through every cell in the body, including the brain, muscles, glands, and skin. As the components of your last meal flow through your bloodstream, they create changes in the function of every organ and in the balance of every body system. The muscle–tension in the walls of the arteries, the levels of vital hormones, the mineral regulation in the kidneys, and thousands of other subtle, but important, balances are all affected by the food you eat. . . .

"These proteins and other substances then actually become your tissues, become YOU. If you are a pregnant woman, these foods and any possible chemical contaminants they contain become your baby."[11]

Can you see from these statements the vital importance of one's diet immediately before and during pregnancy? The same principles hold true once that child is born. The child will literally become the foods he has eaten as he matures.[12] The child may grow up on a diet of primarily raw living plant foods and enjoy sickness–free optimal health, or he may grown up on the SAD and follow the path of his peers to and from the doctor's office and the ultimate onset of chronic degeneration.

It has been said that if you want to change the outcome of anything you must make the appropriate changes, which will affect that outcome. If you keep doing the same things, you'll keep getting the same results. It is imperative that we change the way we fuel the body if we are going to get results that are different from that of the multitudes around us.

Renewing Our Minds

Unfortunately, most people operate with a mindset, a core belief system, or a program that was established in the first few years of life. I would suggest to you that you will have to work at re-programming and that ongoing education, support, and practice will be necessary to establish new programs. In Romans 12:1–2, we are told, *"I beseech you therefore, brethren, by the mercies of God, that ye present your bodies a living sacrifice, holy, acceptable unto God, which is your reasonable service. And be not conformed to this world: but be ye transformed by the renewing of your mind, that ye may prove what is that good, and acceptable, and perfect, will of God."*

Transforming or renewing our minds takes education, support, emotional involvement, and commitment. For most of us, our programming tells us there is nothing wrong with the SAD. When we begin changing our paradigms (renewing our minds), we will find family and friends telling us that what we are doing is not normal. But as you look around at the vast majority of our 'normal' population and see children with colds, flu, juvenile diabetes, cancer, etc., and that 50% of the population is dying from cardiovascular disease, I would ask, "Who wants to be normal?"

It may be important for us to realize that our well-meaning family members and friends can lift us up and support us, or they can bring us down as we strive to institute positive change in our lives. We must be prudent in the advice we follow.

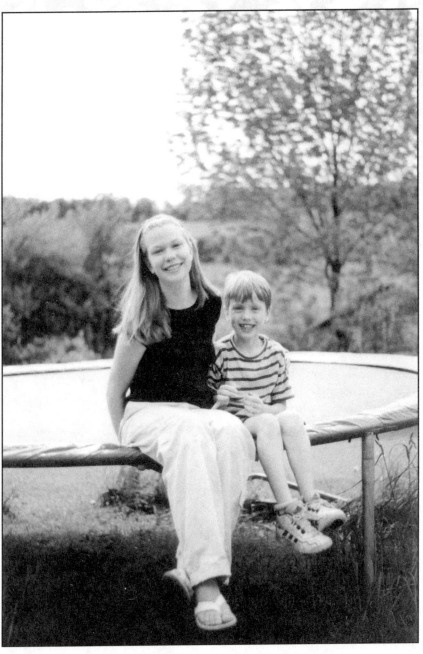

Alexia and Lee Wright—shown here at ages 13 and 8. Raised vegetarian
and since ages 12 and 7 they have eaten only raw foods.

CHAPTER 2

Basic Concept of The Hallelujah Diet®

The basic concept of The Hallelujah Diet® is to eliminate the processed dead foods (the five "killer" foods), namely: meat, dairy products, table salt, white flour, and processed sugars, and then we nourish the body with the living foods as closely to the way nature provides them as possible. A plant–based diet consisting of 75–85% raw foods, freshly extracted vegetable juices, and 15–25% cooked foods has proven to support optimal health.

Internal Toxicity

What does this mean for the couple planning for conception? First of all, they need to be aware of the importance of eliminating the harmful foods, nourishing the body with living foods, and keeping the body clean or detoxified internally.

When a person makes positive dietary and lifestyle changes, they may experience some symptoms of cleansing. It is important that his or her bowels are functioning optimally for rapid and efficient elimination of the toxins. The Hallelujah Diet® currently includes the use of a fiber-based herbal product to initially promote gently cleansing of the colon, to facilitate the removal of the toxins, and to restore optimal bowel activity with two to three good eliminations daily. While this method is ideal for most people, it is not recommended for long–term use or for pregnant or lactating women. This type of product contains numerous herbs that are not intended for long–term use and should not be used by pregnant or lactating women without supervision of a knowledgeable health care professional. It may be wise for women to discontinue its use after conception and while nursing unless directed otherwise by a medical doctor.

An alternative during this period and after the initial cleansing may be a serving of freshly ground organic flaxseed in a cup of organic apple juice or water each morning. It is important that the seed be freshly ground each morning. This may be accomplished in an inexpensive coffee grinder. An average serving varies from a tablespoon to one-fourth cup daily. A quarter cup will provide over 11 grams of fiber, 9,000 mg of Omega 3, and 2,250 mg of Omega 6 essential fats. That's the equivalent of the Omega 3 and Omega 6 found in approximately one and one-half tablespoons of flaxseed oil.

Optimal Nutrition

Once the bowels are functioning well, and you are achieving two to three bowel movements daily with well formed, light colored, soft stools, you can consider the living foods with which you are fueling your body.

The Hallelujah Diet's® 75–85% raw foods and juices, and 15–25% cooked foods, have proven to be an ideal balance in providing the body with a wide variety of nutrients in a synergistic blend that is bio-available to the body. The small percentage of cooked foods allows the body access to those nutrients that are more easily assimilated from cooked foods, such as lycopenes from tomatoes and the increased antioxidant activity of beta carotene found in such foods as cooked carrots. In reality, we have the best of both. The human body is designed by God to receive its nutrients in a bio-available synergistic blend as found in living foods (Genesis 1:29). Nutrients in a living-foods diet are easily assimilated by the body.

Having your own garden is one of the best ways to ensure your foods are chemical free and nutrient dense. For those who cannot or who choose not to maintain a garden, it is important to consume as much local organically grown produce as possible when in season. In this age, when commercial farming has depleted many of the minerals from the soil, it is important that we consume a wide variety of raw foods, preferably grown from various parts of the country and as fresh as possible to ensure a sufficient intake of nutrients.

A study conducted at Rutgers University[13] showed a wide variation of mineral composition of vegetables grown in different parts of the country. Looking at tomatoes for example, levels of calcium ranged from a high of 23 mg to a low of 4.5 mg, while magnesium ranged from a high of 59.2 mg to a low of 4.5 mg depending upon the area of the country in which they were grown. Fortunately, in today's age of mass transportation, we can have produce from all over the world within a few days of harvesting. However, we must keep in mind that fruits are often harvested before they are ripe, thus severely limiting their nutrient content.

While there can be a staggering range of nutrient content in fruits and vegetables, it is wise to keep in mind that the greatest cause of nutrient loss is food manufacturing rather than farming practices. Such items as refined white flour and white rice lose more than 77% of their zinc, chromium, and manganese in the refining process. "More than half the nutrients in the food you eat are destroyed before they reach your plate, depending on the food you choose, how you store it, and how you cook it. Every process that food goes through, whether boiling, baking, frying, or freezing, takes its toll. . . . On an average, 20 – 70% of the nutrient content of leafy vegetables is lost in cooking."[14]

Microwave cooking is by far the most destructive and should be avoided if one desires optimal health. A study published in the November issue of *The Journal of the Science of Food and Agriculture* found that broccoli "zapped" in the microwave with a little water lost up to 97% of the beneficial antioxidant chemicals it contains. By comparison, steamed broccoli lost 11% or fewer of its antioxidants.

Ideally, our fruit consumption should not exceed 15% of our total dietary intake. Fruits are cleansers of the body while the vegetables are the builders. "Generally, vegetables are considered a better source of minerals, while fruit is considered a better source of vitamins. Taking into account the fact that most of the fruit in this country is picked before it is ripe for shipping to market, vegetables would probably be superior on both counts, since unripe fruit is lower in vitamin content."[15] It is also important to keep in mind that many of our fruits are hybrids, containing as much as 30% more sugar than the fruits our ancestors ate.[16]

Essential Fatty Acids

You want to be sure to include a good source of essential fats to your diet—fats that the body cannot manufacture and that must be provided by the diet. During the last trimester, the infant's brain develops very rapidly. An adequate supply of the EFAs (essential fatty acids) is critical at this time. Not only are they vital for optimal brain development, but they are also important for maintaining the structural parts of the cell membranes and in the production of hormone–like substances known as eicosanoids. "Eicosanoids help regulate blood pressure, blood clot formation, blood lipids, and the immune response to injury and infection."[17] We can readily see the important role of these essential fats in the development of a healthy child. **It is vital that they are included in the diet.** Good sources of essential fatty acids are freshly ground flaxseed, flaxseed oil, raw walnuts, Udo's oil, or a good algae–derived DHA (docosahexaenoic acid—an Omega 3 long chain polyunsaturated fatty acid) supplement.

One other area of concern while discussing the importance of EFAs is the crucial role DHA has in the development of the infant and young baby. The human brain consists of approximately 60% structural fat, with DHA being the most abundant component:

"The most significant research on DHA deals with infant brain development. During the late stages of fetal development and immediately following birth, the human brain grows very rapidly. The DHA content of the fetal brain increases three to five times during the final trimester of pregnancy and triples yet again during the first 12 weeks of life."[18]

DHA is also important in the development of the eye, as it is the most abundant fat in the retina. "To assure their babies have enough DHA, pregnant and nursing women may want to consider taking DHA supplements. . . . Studies show that DHA supplementation of pregnant and lactating women increases DHA available to the fetus and the nursing baby."[19]

It is well-known that breastfed infants develop with a slightly higher IQ, 3–6 points higher, than non-breastfed infants. The DHA content of mother's milk is thought to contribute greatly to this. Dr. James Anderson tells us that in the U.S.: "The DHA content in breast milk has gone down 67% in the last 60 years. The DHA levels in breast milk of American women are 50% less than those of European women, and about 66% less than those of Japanese women."[20] While the adult body can synthesize small amounts of DHA if the Omega 3 fats are available, pregnant vegan women may not be able to synthesize adequate amounts to optimally meet the needs of the growing fetus. There are no good dietary plant-based sources of this essential nutrient other that sea algae.

It is fairly common for most people on the SAD to get an excess of Omega 6 fatty acid while being deficient in Omega 3 fatty acid. "It has been estimated that 60% of the population gets too much of one essential fatty acid, and that 95% of the population gets too little of the other."[21] When we move to a primarily raw plant-based diet, we want to ensure we are getting our EFAs in the necessary quantity, as well as the proper ratio. This is vitally important for pregnant and nursing women. Many women ensure this need is met by incorporating 2–3 tablespoons of freshly ground organic flaxseed (great added to a fruit smoothie), or 1–2 tablespoons of flaxseed oil or Udo's Choice Perfected Oil Blend into their diet on a daily basis. Udo's oil has been specially blended to yield a 2 to 1 ratio of Omega 3 to Omega 6 fats, thought to be an ideal ratio for the human body. Either of these oils can also be used to make an excellent salad dressing by combining it with a little fresh lemon juice and herbs. Udo's Oil can also be added to a baked potato after it is split (rather than butter) or on a piece of sprouted whole grain toast. There is a host of ways to work these forms of EFAs into your diet.

Good sources rich in the essential Omega 3 fatty acid are flaxseed oil and freshly ground flaxseed. A serving of 1–3 tablespoons of freshly ground flaxseed (grind fresh each day in a coffee grinder) is an excellent source of fiber as well as essential fats. Chia seeds, although not as readily available, are also rich in Omega 3.

If a pregnant woman is lacking in the correct fatty acids, the body uses less desirable fatty acids. This may result in less than optimal brain development in the fetus, as well as further depletion of the mother's essential fatty acid stores.

Vitamin B-12

Along with the consideration of EFAs, it is also important for one (and not just those who avoid animal products) to be sure there is an adequate source of B-12 in the diet. It is vital that the body's B-12 needs are met. Vitamin B-12 is important for maintaining the myelin sheath that surrounds and protects the nerve fibers, as well as for normal blood cell growth. A deficiency in this area may result in anemia or neurological problems. To ensure the mother's health and that of the developing fetus, it is important to be sure there is adequate B-12 in her diet.

Michael Donaldson, Ph.D., researcher for the Hallelujah Acres® Foundation, has pointed out that a B-12 deficiency can be a common occurrence but is extremely easy to avoid by simply adding a small amount of a good B-12 supplement to the diet two or three times weekly. In his research, he determined the best method of testing for a B-12 deficiency to be a simple urine assay for methylmalonic acid. This urine assay can be handled through the mail by a reputable laboratory. "The urinary MMA assay is very specific for B-12 and much more reliable than a serum B-12 assay."[22] A sublingual methylcobalamin supplement is the best method to be sure of obtaining a sufficient supply of B-12. According to Dr. Donaldson, one-half of a caplet twice a week should be adequate to ensure no B-12 deficiency develops for a healthy adult. The body's need for B-12 is very minimal, yet vital.

Not only is vitamin B-12 a vital nutrient for pregnant and nursing women, but, research is confirming the benefits of a B-12, B-6, and Folic Acid combination in regards to lowering homocysteine levels in the body. Evidence suggests that elevated levels of homocysteine may be an underlying cause of cardiovascular disease and an independent risk factor for heart attack, stroke, and peripheral vascular disease.

A discussion of vitamin B-12 would be incomplete without looking briefly at the role our intestinal flora plays in the production and utilization of our B vitamins.

Probiotics

Some have asked why we would need a B–12 supplement if we are following a diet based on Genesis 1:29. In the Garden of Eden and even up until the last few decades, mankind ate most of his raw foods just the way nature prepared them. They were not contaminated with chemicals, and our ancestors were not overly concerned with washing and sanitizing them. They had some friendly bacteria on them that helped keep our intestinal flora in proper balance. We now know what a critical role our friendly flora plays in our overall quality of health. One of the primary contributions our intestinal flora makes to optimal health is the production of B vitamins, especially vitamin B–12. Unfortunately, the diet and lifestyle we live today is conducive to destroying our friendly flora rather than supporting an optimal balance throughout the gastrointestinal tract. Simply put, many of us do not have adequate intestinal flora to produce adequate levels of vitamin B–12 and must rely on supplementation.

The human gastrointestinal tract is inhabited by an incredibly complex variety of four hundred to five hundred species of micro–flora that coexist in harmony as long as the proper balance is maintained. If this symbiotic relationship is broken due to an imbalance with the friendly flora, the unfriendly flora become parasitic and contribute to a host of problems by interfering with digestion and/or damaging the lining of the intestines. Candida, thrush, fungal overgrowth, and diarrhea are just a few commonly reported symptoms of an imbalance in intestinal flora. It is becoming more evident from recent research and studies that a proper balance in intestinal flora is a critical key to optimal immune function.

It is important for us to realize that antibiotics can have a negative impact on our intestinal flora. Antibiotics typically come in the form of medication, but may also be ingested from the consumption of animal products. Drinking and bathing in chlorinated water, drinking carbonated beverages, eating a diet high in protein, sugar, and fat, as well as a whole host of other dietary and lifestyle factors may lead to a condition called dysbiosis, an imbalance of bacterial flora in the gastrointestinal tract.

Vitamin D

Vitamin D plays an important role in calcium absorption and utilization. Although maternal deficiency is unlikely, it is important to be aware that a severe deficiency in vitamin D may interfere with normal calcium metabolism, resulting in rickets in the fetus. Supplementation is normally not recommended because of the associated toxicity risk with fat–soluble vitamins that are stored in the body.[23] However, it is important for pregnant women in northern climates with little sun exposure to be aware of the possible need of supplementation. **Supplementation with vitamin D should not exceed the upper limit of 2,000 IU per day for adults without the guidance of your health care professional since excess vitamin D is toxic and can produce fetal deformities.**

Vitamin D is unusual in that it fits the classic definition of a hormone— a compound made in one part of the body that travels to another part of the body to exert its effects. We can make all the vitamin D we need through adequate sun exposure. In *The Vegetarian Way* Messina states:

> "Studies indicate that the average light–skinned adult can make adequate vitamin D with ten to fifteen minutes of sun exposure on the hands and face two to three times per week during the summer. Because we store vitamin D, the vitamin we make during the summer can last us through the winter months."[24]

It is important to keep in mind that the darker your skin, the more sun exposure you need. It may take as much as six times more sun exposure to make the same amount of this vitamin in some African Americans as it does in Caucasians. This should be noted when considering a possible need for supplementation.

Once the baby is born, it is important to give him reasonable exposure to sunshine to enhance the production of vitamin D. Unfortunately, sunshine through a glass window does not expose the skin to the ultraviolet rays that are necessary for the production of vitamin D. In areas of limited sunlight, it may be necessary to provide supplemental vitamin D.

Folic Acid or Folate

Along with B-12, it is important to include adequate sources of folic acid. Good dietary sources of folic acid are green leafy vegetables (these can be added to carrot juice), nutritional yeast, brown rice, legumes, lentils, root vegetables, whole grains, and dates. Vegans typically exceed the 1 mg daily requirement.[25] It is important to know that a folate deficiency can impair cell division and protein synthesis, both of which are vital to growing tissue. ". . . [T]wo of the first symptoms of folate deficiency are anemia and GI tract deterioration. . . . Of all vitamins, folate appears to be the most vulnerable to interaction with drugs, which can lead to a secondary deficiency."[26] Adequate folate intake is also important in reducing the risk of neural tube defects.

As we look at the nutritional needs of the body, it becomes increasingly evident how vital the concepts of The Hallelujah Diet® are in maintaining optimal health. Eliminating the harmful elements from one's diet is important. This includes items such as the five "killer" foods, all drugs—including caffeine, over-the-counter drugs, and as many legally prescribed drugs as possible. It is best to obtain nutrients in a synergistic blend from raw foods so that all of the nutrients required for optimal assimilation are available to mother and child.

Protein

Protein plays a vital role in overall health, as well as in the development of the fetus. Fortunately, obtaining adequate protein is not a major concern since most pregnant women in the United States typically exceed the body's required amount of protein. "Pregnant vegetarian women who meet their energy needs by eating ample servings of protein-containing plant foods such as legumes, whole grains, nuts and seeds meet their protein needs as well."[27]

Many of our green foods are rich sources of protein and provide a broad spectrum of vitamins, minerals, and other nutrients necessary for optimal health. Green foods should be used liberally, both raw and cooked, in an optimal diet. A well-rounded plant-based diet is nutrient dense while being low in calories. If adequate calories are consumed to meet the metabolic needs of the body, as well as the energy needs, the protein needs will be met.

Calories

There is little, if any, increase in calorie needs during the first three months of pregnancy. Normally, the second and third trimesters will require about 300 additional calories daily. During lactation, the additional calorie needs may be as much as 500 additional calories daily. Small frequent meals are an excellent way to ensure these needs are met. Raw nuts and seeds, nut and seed butters, avocados, dried fruits, and added fats such as freshly ground flaxseed can provide concentrated calories without bulk. These additional calories will help ensure an adequate amount of protein in the diet.

Calcium

Where will I get my calcium? This is an area of concern for many people, not just pregnant women, when dairy products are eliminated from the diet. After all, the nutritional needs of the skeletal structure of a growing fetus must be met. "About thirty grams—or one ounce—of calcium are deposited in a fetus' bones during pregnancy, most of it during the third trimester."[28] This relatively small calcium need is easily met from a primarily raw plant–based diet. Some of the many calcium–rich foods are: collard, mustard, and turnip greens, as well as kale, broccoli, almonds, and figs.

It is important to realize that a diet moderate in protein intake and devoid of animal products results in a relatively lower calcium requirement. When a primarily raw plant–based diet is maintained, it is much easier for the body to maintain its alkaline pH balance. A predominately alkaline diet allows the body to maintain its calcium reserves, resulting in a need for less dietary calcium intake. It's interesting to observe how an animal in nature such as a cow, which lives exclusively on green grasses and hay, can give birth to a normal, healthy calf with no calcium (or other nutrient) deficiency, and it nurses that calf exclusively on the mother's milk, just as nature intended.

It is extremely difficult to meet the body's calcium needs on a diet based on animal products and processed foods. Not only is this diet low in usable calcium, but it also leaves an acid ash in the body. This acid ash causes the body to leech calcium from the bones in order to maintain the critical alkaline blood pH that is required. The excess calcium that is left over is ultimately eliminated through the urine, resulting in a negative calcium balance and a dramatic decrease in bone density.

Iron

Iron needs during pregnancy are increased since both the infant and the mother are busy creating new blood. Because of the extra iron needed to support the increased blood volume, as well as that required by the placenta and fetus, it is important that daily requirements are met through the mother's diet. Iron is essential in the production of healthy blood cells that carry oxygen from the lungs to the rest of the body. To ensure that the mother has a good iron supply and that the baby will, in turn, have an optimal iron supply at birth, it is important that mother include a significant amount of iron–rich foods in the diet.

> **Testimony:** From Florida, Allie Olsen's testimony is indicative of how a pregnant woman's nutritional needs are met on The Hallelujah Diet®. *"Our first son, Benjamin, was born January 25, 1999. My pregnancy was good, and I considered my delivery to be pretty good at the time. We had a conventional birth in the hospital, and I was given pitosin, an epidural, and an episiotomy to 'help my body' do this otherwise natural thing. Throughout my pregnancy, I was anemic, even though I took prenatal vitamins with extra iron. I was on the Standard American Diet.*

> *"Shortly after his birth, our family made the switch. We started following the Hallelujah lifestyle after my dad had a heart attack at 49. I am only 21, so my husband and I didn't have significant changes other than weight loss. . . . but my father has!! Anyways, we have been on the diet for about two years now and are pregnant with our second child. We are doing things more naturally this time. We have decided to have a home birth, and I have not been supplementing my diet with prenatal vitamins. I had to go for routine blood tests, and I'm SO EXCITED about the results! I am not anemic this*

time! Isn't that exactly opposite of what SHOULD have happened according to the world's wisdom? But praise God, all (yes, I said ALL—including protein and calcium) my levels are normal even though I don't take supplements or consume meat/dairy! I think this is definitely a HALLELUJAH kind of testimony!"

Dr. Klaper points out that " . . . one thing is apparent: eating red meat is no insurance against developing anemia (too little red blood), as most pregnant (and non–pregnant) women who develop iron deficiency anemia eat red meat! They also may be drinking cow's milk and eating dairy products, both of which have been shown to inhibit the absorption of iron."[29]

Good sources of iron are: green leafy vegetables (organically grown lettuces, etc., may be juiced with the carrots), whole grains (both sprouted and cooked), beets (root and greens may be juiced with carrots), lima beans, lentils, almonds, peaches, pears, dried prunes, raisins, and sea vegetables. Interestingly enough, vitamin C markedly increases the absorption of iron from food into the body. Green leafy vegetables contain both vitamin C and iron. Combining vitamin C rich foods (turnip greens, broccoli, Brussels sprouts, sweet potatoes, peppers, tomatoes, and cabbage) with our iron rich foods can help increase iron absorption.

Testimony: Carrie Malkmus, from North Carolina, writes: *"The first trimester was the toughest part of the pregnancy. My major complaint was not wanting to eat; I had no appetite. During that time, I did manage to consume 6–8 tablespoons of dehydrated barley juice powder along with a couple glasses of carrot juice almost every day. My appetite greatly increased once I passed week fourteen.*

"The rest of the pregnancy went great! My hemoglobin levels (indicator of iron status) stayed at the high end of the normal range until the last month of the pregnancy when it dropped a few points—still within the normal range. I had virtually no edema, just a minimal amount of swelling in my fingers in the last week or so of the pregnancy.

"My weight gain was slow and gradual. I gained a total of 27 pounds and got zero stretch marks from it!

"I used dehydrated barley juice powder (6–8 Tbsp/day) as my prenatal vitamin. I consumed a modified version of the Hallelujah Diet—30% cooked overall (some days more, some days less, depending on my appetite) and I ate breakfast. My breakfast consisted of a fruit smoothie, fruit salad, oatmeal, or another whole grain cereal.

"The labor was not the painless experience I had prayed for. However, the midwives did comment that it was one of the most peaceful first births they had ever seen. Dylan Alexander Malkmus was 6 pounds even and 20 ¼ inches long and very healthy and alert.

"I believe that the Hallelujah Diet helped me control my weight gain, helped my energy level, and provided the nutrients and enzymes that Dylan and I needed to have such a healthy pregnancy, delivery, and baby."

"Regardless of the nutritional state of the mother, there is another prophylactic procedure which should be carried out in order to assure the infant has his rightful supply of iron. This procedure consists of allowing the umbilical cord to cease pulsating prior to its severance following delivery. This measure will increase the infant's blood supply by about 100cc and will thereby add about 45mg of iron to the body's iron stores. The importance of this procedure can be appreciated when it is realized that this amount of iron is about twice the amount which the average infant retains during the entire first six months of life . . ."[30] We need to be aware that the developing fetus draws on the mother's iron stores to create stores of its own to last through the first four to six months of life, since mother's milk, which is the exclusive diet, is not a rich source of iron.

It is interesting that nature makes provisions for this increased need for iron by the cessation of menstruation, the major route of iron loss in women; during pregnancy; and by the body's increased ability (almost tripled) to absorb iron due to an increase in blood transferring the body's iron–absorbing and iron–carrying protein.

Premature infants and those not carried to full term may be in need of additional iron sources. This should be determined with the help of your health care professional.

While the scope of this book will not allow us to examine each individual vitamin and mineral requirement of the body, we have touched on some of the major areas of concern for pregnant women. This should provide convincing evidence that the body is well able to meets the nutrient needs to support a healthy pregnancy on a primarily raw vegan diet. It is important that a pregnant woman take into consideration the increased needs for various vitamin, minerals, proteins, and fats, and that she ensure she is eating adequate amounts of the foods that meet these needs. For a more in–depth analysis of the overall dietary needs, a study of the various books referenced in the bibliography section will prove fruitful.

> **Testimony:** Nicole Nixon continues, *"Being pregnant (creating a new life) and nursing causes the body to burn up energy, enzymes, and nutrients at a much more rapid pace than another person's body who is not pregnant or nursing. Most of the time, I eat twice as much as everyone else before I feel satisfied. For example, it takes two apples, not one, to satisfy me. At dinner, I have two helpings of salad and two baked potatoes or two bowls of rice or more before I feel full. What I am trying to say is when you are pregnant or nursing you really are eating for two. You are creating a life, a living being. Your body needs living food with enzymes, vitamins, and minerals to support itself and then it needs more on top of that to create a new life. Please don't feel like something is wrong, and especially don't feel guilty for needing to eat more. But please make wise choices about the food you choose. Every time you eat, you are ingesting the building blocks that your child will be made of."*

CHAPTER 3

Birthing Options

*And he said, "When ye do the office of a midwife to the
Hebrew women, and see them upon the stools ... And the
midwives said unto Pharaoh, Because the Hebrew women
are not as the Egyptian women; for they are lively, and are
delivered ere the midwives come in unto them."*
—*Exodus 1:16a, 19*

Long before the anticipated delivery date, and perhaps even before
the pregnancy takes place, there are many factors to consider and
decisions to be made. Not the least of these is the decision as
to where the birth will take place. May I suggest that a great deal of
thought go into making this decision? I would encourage you to do
your homework early on and make the preparations to follow through
with your convictions based on what you learn.

While the vast majority of babies are born in hospital settings today, if
we look back through history, we see this is definitely not the norm and
may not be the most desirable setting. Lewis Mehl, M.D., conducted a
study about the safety of homebirths:

> "The study found that women birthing in hospitals were five
> times more likely to have high blood pressure during labor; nine
> times more likely to tear; three times more likely to hemorrhage;
> and three times more likely to undergo cesarean section. . . .

> "The hospital–born babies were six times more likely to suffer
> fetal distress before birth; four times more likely to need
> assistance to start breathing; and four times more likely to
> develop infections. . . .

"In every single category of comparison, home birth mothers and infants did vastly better. While 30 of the infants born in hospitals suffered birth injuries, not a single one of the infants born at home suffered this fate."[31]

A more natural setting that many women are choosing today is a home birth assisted by a midwife. The testimonies from women following a natural plant–based diet and experiencing a home birth are remarkable.

Testimony: Danette Gentry, from California, writes, *"Baby Grace and I just finished our first year as a nursing couple on the Hallelujah Diet. Grace was exclusively nursed (no supplements, juice, or water of any kind) the first six months. When she began to show interest in solid foods, she began sampling off my vegan plate (no canned baby foods).*

"She still nurses on demand at one year of age, and along with her two older sisters, enjoys fresh squeezed orange juice and carrot juice each day.

"Her disposition is one of the most remarkable I have ever seen. She is the sweetest, most patient baby, content and peaceful. I named her Grace as she made me praise the grace of God to behold such a beautiful spirited child!

"Grace came into the world through a drugless home birth, bright–eyed, beautiful and big (9 lbs. 12 oz.)—without a tear, scratch, or even bruise to her mom. I attribute this to asking the Lord specifically for a peaceful and safe delivery with no tearing, and being open to what He directed in my prenatal care—including a vegan diet—and WOW, did He deliver!

"As a mom over 40, the Hallelujah Diet helped me recover much faster than I had with my second baby at age 38. The carrot juice and dehydrated barley juice powder helped me get my energy back. Whenever I felt foggy, I would juice some more carrots for the boost my body needed, as the hormones adjusted from pregnancy to nursing.

"After the birth of Grace, and fully on the Hallelujah Diet, I returned to my pre–pregnancy weight rapidly. I am so thankful I was able to

resume my responsibilities at home and to care for my other children so much faster than with my previous births. Nursing has been great and Grace is strong and took her first step at eight months. As I write this, I am truly humbled and thankful for my healthy baby and the knowledge that has been revealed to us."

Here in the United States, where physicians oversee 95% of all births, most women assume that the hospital is the place for the delivery and that a medical doctor will be in charge. Our society has for years trained us in this mindset. Seldom do women even realize there are other options. Yet, might I suggest even better options?

It might be a good idea, even before getting pregnant, to talk with other mothers concerning their experience with childbirth. Where did the birth take place? Who was in charge of the situation? Were their wishes honored? What would they do differently if they had other options in the future?

"In the United States, physicians oversee 95% of all births. In Europe, where infant mortality rates are superior to ours, midwives (non–physicians, almost always women, skilled in the art and science of birthing) attend 75% of births. In every single one of the nations where infant mortality rates are lower than ours, midwives are the principal birth attendants."[32]

Unfortunately, like disease care, childbirth is big business. Hospitals and doctors, eager to get their share of money spent on childbirth, are not eager to let potential mothers consider other options. Midwives have been persecuted since the sixteenth century in Europe. John Robbins' book *Reclaiming Our Health* has an eye–opening chapter entitled "A Modern–Day Witch–Hunt," which traces some of the opposition to and persecution of midwives up to our present day.

In recent years we have begun seeing a more relaxed attitude from the traditional medical community toward alternatives in childbirth, as well as various alternative approaches to wellness. A high percentage of the U.S. population now seeks alternative treatments, as it has become quite evident that the traditional medical establishment is unable to cure any disease.

Birthing Centers

According to John Robbins, in 1975 there were only five freestanding birthing centers in the United States. By 1994, the number had grown to 140 with an additional 60 planned. These non–hospital centers provide an atmosphere where births can take place in a normal and healthy environment without the mother–to–be being required to fit into the normal rigid hospital routine. They have the freedom to move around at leisure and choose any position they desire for labor. Interference with the process is minimal. The soon–to–be mother is in charge and the birthing process is assisted by a trained and competent midwife.[33]

In 1989, the *New England Journal of Medicine* published the results of the largest study ever done on freestanding birthing centers. "The infant death rate for all births begun at birth centers (including breech births, twins, and those that got into trouble and had to be transferred to hospitals) was much lower than that for births occurring in hospitals. . . . The cesarean rate was 4.4%, less than one–fifth the typical hospital average."[34] Satisfaction with the experience was so great that 99% said they would recommend this type of facility to friends. The costs were also significantly less."

The track record of midwife–attended births far outshines that of the medical profession in the hospital setting. The long–term benefits to mother and child are overwhelming. Researcher David Stewart "estimates that if all American women had birth attendants with a midwife approach, mother and baby mortality would be halved, and the rates of brain–damaged children and other birth injuries and complications in newborns would be cut by three–quarters. Other authorities agree, adding that we'd save $8.5 billion a year."[35]

> **Testimony:** Carrie Malkmus continues: "*We had Dylan at a maternity center, which is run by certified nurse midwives and is just a few minutes away from a hospital. This is where baby #2 will be born as well.*"

Home Births

While in the past mothers choosing a homebirth assisted by a midwife were often ridiculed, today they are looked upon with more respect.

People are realizing that the typical mindset may not be the best, and that they must take charge of their health rather than depend upon someone else to do what is best for them. Many women today are taking charge of their health and pregnancies while going against the traditional mainstream thinking. Like the increasing use of birthing centers, homebirths are on the rise also.

In rural Tennessee there is a community known simply as The Farm. In the 1970s and 1980s, more that 1,700 babies were born at home there, all attended by midwives. Statistics for these births were nothing short of spectacular. Interventions were almost nonexistent. Forceps were used in less than one in every 200 births (compared to one in every two births in some hospitals). Some 98% of the women gave birth without any drugs (while in many U.S. hospitals most women are drugged). Even twins and breech presentations were usually successfully delivered at home. The cesarean rate was less than 2%. Despite taking on high–risk situations, the neonatal mortality rate was far lower than the average American hospital.[36]

The safety aspect of home births and that of freestanding birthing centers is by far superior to that of hospital births for the mother as well as the infant. Various studies have demonstrated that the infant mortality rate for home births is far lower than that of hospital deliveries. In commenting on researcher David Stewart's work in this area, John Robbins states, "The evidence testifying that maternity systems based on midwifery have better baby and mother outcomes is overwhelming. 'The database for these figures is in the millions, is global in scope, and spans almost a century, up to and including the present,' says Stewart."[37]

Another area of concern for pregnant women is the abnormally high rate of cesarean sections in this country. As John Robbins points out, as the rate of cesarean sections soared, our ranking in infant mortality among other nations dropped dramatically. Infants delivered in this manner are more likely to suffer respiratory problems and distress. A Finnish study of 8,088 children, followed since birth, shows that children whose birth was accompanied by special obstetric procedures were at significantly greater risk of developing asthma.[38] The risk of infection, hemorrhage, and even death are many times greater in a cesarean delivery than in a vaginal delivery. Avoiding medical intervention (as much as possible) during childbirth usually results in much healthier children. You simply cannot improve on God's design.

We could look at research studies and statistics that, one right after the other, point to the overall superiority of choosing a birthing place other than a local hospital. While I am not opposed to hospitals and the vital role doctors play in traumatic injury, I think women should realize that they have the right to choose an environment of peace and dignity where the entire birthing process can unfold naturally and unrushed. They should be allowed to give utmost consideration to the safety and well-being of their baby, as well as themselves, as they make this an informed decision. I would encourage each couple to read John Robbins' book *Reclaiming Our Health*, as well as other resources that discuss the birthing options.

Testimony: Mrs. Pavelka writes, *"Our entire family adopted the Hallelujah Diet three years ago. Our first child is almost five, so she was almost two when we started on the Hallelujah Diet. Our second child is three and was a nursing infant when we changed lifestyles. Our third child is eighteen months old and has been 'grown' totally on the Hallelujah Diet. There is a difference in children who are 'made' on the Hallelujah Diet from conception vs. those who come into it after weaning. Out of all of them, the oldest has the weakest immune system and is the only one who has ever been to a doctor.*

"As far as the birth story is concerned, baby number three (our Hallelujah Baby) was born at home, as were the other two, but this was a much easier delivery—two pushes and she was out. It just happened that the midwife couldn't be with us, so my husband and I delivered alone. I made supper for the family, Dad bathed and put the children to bed at 8:30, and the baby was born at 9:30 P.M. Active labor had started after my afternoon nap, but I kept busy with the normal routine, getting clothes in from the line, sweeping the porch, and just rocking on all fours when necessary. At one point my son asked, 'Mommy, what are you looking for?' The baby was born in excellent health, great color, no mucus on her body, great lungs, alert, and she nursed immediately. I wouldn't go back to eating the Standard American Diet for anything. I feel so much different, our health is so much better, and I can see the 'proof' daily before my eyes."

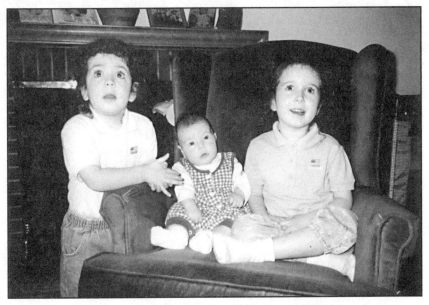

Abby, Kelly and Emily McGovern—all three healthy, happy, *Hallelujah Babies.*

CHAPTER 4

Getting Off to the Right Start

Blessed is the womb that bare thee, and the paps
which thou hast sucked.
—Luke 11:27

Now that the nine months' journey of pregnancy has culminated in the birth of a healthy baby, where do we go from here? For the past nine months, baby has been in that warm snug environment listening to the rhythmic sounds of mother's internal environment. Suddenly, he or she is thrust into unfamiliar surroundings. There are many physical, mental, spiritual, and emotional, as well as nutritional, needs to be met. I would encourage you to seek out resources that address these issues so that you will be better equipped to handle them.

Breastfeeding

There is no question that the ideal nourishment for a baby is the milk produced by the mother who gave birth to that baby. As early as the sixteenth week of pregnancy, changes begin to occur in the mother's breast in preparation for producing the perfect food for the developing infant. There is no way we can address this issue as thoroughly as it should be addressed in the space we can devote to it here. Entire books have been written on this subject. We'll simply center in on a few vital issues in hopes that it will inspire the young mother–to–be to more fully investigate the innumerable benefits to both mother and child.

Breastfeeding is certainly the best, most natural form of nutrition during the infant's first year of life, and holds great benefit for the mother as well. Breastmilk not only contains nutrients, but also antibodies that bolster the baby's immune system. Very importantly, the breastfeeding years create emotional security in the child through the many hours of intimate contact with the mother. The breastmilk of vegan mothers also provides a measure of safety for the baby. Nursing women who eat the conventional animal–based American diet consume meat, dairy products, and fish that contain chemical contaminants such as hormones, antibiotics, and pesticides, which fail to provide that measure of assurance.

> "These substances are then secreted into the woman's breastmilk. During its first year, the baby is still developing its brain, endocrine glands, and other vital tissues—and thus is vulnerable to even small amounts of these potent chemicals. Vegan women who do not eat animal products secrete far less of these contaminants into their breast milk than flesh and dairy–eating women. Thus, vegan infants are spared a potentially serious chemical assault early in life."[39]

A report from the Union of Concerned Scientists stated that 25 million pounds, or roughly 70% of total U.S. antibiotic production, are fed to chickens, pigs, and cows for non–therapeutic purposes like growth promotion.[40] Is it any wonder we are seeing an alarming increase in antibiotic resistance?

It is vital for the lactating mother to ensure her diet contains optimal nutrients and that those "foods" that negatively impact the health of the nursing infant be eliminated. Stacelynn Caughlan states:

> "Within hours of a meal, the type of fat consumed is the predominant fat in milk. This means you must be aware of what to eat—and not eat! During the prenatal and neonatal stages, fat is the one substance that plays an important role in growth, neurological development and function and learning and behavior. . . . Breastmilk is a very rich source of Essential Fatty Acids (EFAs), but only if the mother's dietary consumption is adequate. If your diet is high in trans–fatty acids, these too will be passed on to the infant.

"Trans–fatty acids are found in hydrogenated oils and processed foods and have been linked to cardiovascular risk, neurological underdevelopment, and other lifelong risks in children. Even if the diet is rich in EFAs, the inclusion of trans–fats will prohibit their metabolization. Neither you nor your baby will receive all possible benefits."[41]

We would do well to remember that the infant, through the breastmilk, would also take in any drugs such as alcohol and caffeine consumed by the mother. These drugs may impair the immature liver of the infant.

Some researchers believe the Omega 3 fats are so essential that a deficiency on the part of the mother and infant can impair the development of the child's immune system and nervous system to the extent that the child could have a lifetime of emotional, learning, and immune system disorders.

It is estimated that 75–80% of all two–month–old babies are bottle–fed. Could we be seeing the effects of decades of Omega 3 deficiencies in mothers and infants manifest in such rampant illnesses as chronic ear infections, nose and throat infections, allergies, candida, hyperactivity, ADD and ADHD, and autistic behavior?

According to John Finnegan, researchers at the Mayo Clinic suggest that this important fat be supplemented in every pregnancy, and that refined and hydrogenated fats be avoided in this critical period.[42] It is important that pregnant as well as nursing mothers make sure they have an adequate intake of EFAs. One way of doing so is to include two to three tablespoons of freshly ground organic flaxseed in the diet each day. An algae derived DHA supplement included daily as well will help insure this vital nutrient is present for optimal brain and visual development.

Growth is faster during the first six months of life than at any other time during the life cycle. The nutrients the infant receives during these first six months will have a major impact on the long–term health of the child. At no other time in life will the baby have the same need for fats, proteins, and a vast array of other macro and micro nutrients, all of which are supplied in ideal quantities in breastmilk. Breastmilk contains everything (if Mom is on an optimal diet!) that the baby needs in order to enjoy optimal health and reach maximum potential. This should be the exclusive diet of the infant for at least the first six months. There should be no need for supplements of any kind for an infant who is thriving on a diet of breastmilk.

Dr. Jack Newman points out some areas to consider in helping the new mother and baby get off to the right start. He suggests that the baby be put to the mother's breast as soon after delivery as possible, at least within the first fifteen to thirty minutes. This is an excellent time for bonding and should not be a time when the infant is forced to nurse, but rather allowed to proceed at its own pace.[43]

There may be times when an infant simply needs oral gratification rather than nursing strictly for food. There should be no restriction on feeding time or frequency. Proper positioning and latching on is critical. A mother would do well to become educated in these areas prior to the delivery.

Often there is concern over the possibility of mother not producing enough milk. Usually this concern comes from misconceptions concerning the baby's behavior and/or weight gain. It is rare that the mother cannot produce enough milk. Maintaining a diet rich in freshly extracted vegetable juices, an abundance of fresh green leafy vegetables, fruits, and a good balance of whole grains, legumes, and raw nuts and seeds should ensure an ample supply of high quality breast milk. It is important to keep in mind that mother's nutritional needs are significantly higher as she is eating for two. As mentioned earlier, snacking or eating small frequent meals is a good way to ensure the additional calorie intake is achieved.

It is common for infants of vegetarian families to grow at a slightly slower and more optimal rate than that of formula fed infants or infants of mothers on the SAD. It is also normal for the baby to lose a little weight the first few days, but by ten days of age that weight is normally regained. Sometimes as early as day four or five, an infant may be over his or her birth weight. For the first two months, an infant can be expected to gain about an ounce per day and about ½ ounce per day the next four months. After the age of six months, the growth rate will slow significantly.

Various studies indicate that breastfed babies excel in intelligence and cognitive development, with normal development of jaw and facial muscles, and they are less likely to be afflicted with respiratory illness, ear infections, gastrointestinal infections and diseases, childhood cancer, diabetes, and sudden infant death syndrome than babies fed otherwise.

The immunological protection offered to the infant through breastfeeding is unsurpassed and is extremely valuable during the first year while the infant's immune system is developing.

"During the first two or three days after delivery, the breasts produce colostrum, a premilk substance containing mostly serum with antibodies and white blood cells. Colostrum (like breast milk) helps protect the newborn from infections against which the mother has developed immunity. The maternal antibodies swallowed with the milk inactivate disease–causing bacteria within the digestive tract before they can start infections. This explains, in part, why breastfed infants have fewer intestinal infections than formula–fed infants."[44]

Colostrum is one of the most, if not the most, important foods an infant will ever ingest. This early milk is thicker and stickier than the regular breast milk will be in a few days. Likewise, the nutrient make–up is different. Not only does it contain all of the essential amino acids, but it is also higher in overall protein, vitamins A and E, and minerals such as potassium and sodium.

Colostrum is vitally important during the first few hours and days, even in very small amounts. Initially, it will act as a laxative as it stimulates the passing of the meconium, the infant's first stool. Since colostrum is readily digested, it helps stabilize the infant's blood sugar, as well as provides protection for the sensitive lining of the gastrointestinal tract, and helps create a barrier to ward off infections. During the next two weeks, the amount of colostrum in the regular breast milk will gradually taper off.

"In addition to antibodies and colostrum, breast milk provides other powerful agents that help to fight against bacterial infection. Among them are bifidus factors, which favor the growth of the 'friendly' bacterium *Lactobacillus bifidus* in the infant's digestive tract so that other harmful bacteria cannot gain a foothold there. An iron–binding protein in breast milk, lactoferrin, keeps unfriendly bacteria from getting the iron they need to grow, helps absorb iron into the infant's bloodstream, and kills some bacteria directly. Also present is a growth factor that stimulates the development and maintenance of the infant's digestive tract and its protective factors. Several breast milk enzymes such as lipase also help protect the infant against infection. Clearly, breast milk is a very special substance."[45]

As mentioned earlier, breastfeeding offers exceptional benefits to the mother as well as to the infant. Breastfeeding mothers recover from the birthing process more rapidly as the uterus is encouraged to contract normally and the amount of blood loss is reduced. Breastfeeding also reduces the risk of the mother developing breast cancer. "[T]he greater the total months of breastfeeding, the lower the risk of developing cancer."[46] Simply realizing that for every month a mother breastfeeds her baby her risk of getting breast cancer is going down should provide ample encouragement for a mother to nurse her baby for an extended period of time.

Many mothers nurse their baby for up to 24 months or longer. They realize that the benefits her milk provides in building the baby's immunity are continuing, although he is nursing much less frequently. As the frequency of nursing lessens, the milk increases the concentration of protective factors. This is a strong indication that babies are designed to ideally nurse longer than a year. It is interesting that the American Academy of Pediatricians now recommends nursing for at least a year.

Alternatives to Breastfeeding

While breastfeeding is the ideal, there may be some situations (although rare) when breastfeeding is not an option. All possible options for breastfeeding should be exhausted before a mother resorts to any other option. The potential benefits to both mother and child are too great to give this passing consideration. It is impossible for any other option to equal the benefits of breastfeeding, and the long–term implications justify taking the necessary steps to ensure your infant has the best start in life possible.

Since there is not an ideal substitute for breastfeeding, if mother simply cannot breastfeed her infant, the next best option would be to extract her milk and make that available for the baby. It isn't uncommon for mothers to exclusively breastfeed their baby for the first two or three months and find they need to supplement the breastfeeding for one or more of many reasons. The next best option to breastfeeding would be to pump mother's milk and to store it in the refrigerator for later use.

If for some reason mother's milk is not an option, a breastmilk bank should not be forgotten.

There is one downside with using milk from a breastmilk bank: to ensure the safety of the milk supply, the milk is pasteurized. This would destroy the enzyme activity in the milk and alter the chemical makeup to some extent, but the end product would be a superior choice to that of a man–made scientific formula product. There are several breastmilk banks across the country. A check with the local hospital may prove fruitful. Dr. Newman's book *The Ultimate Breastfeeding Book of Answers* offers a listing of some of these in the resource section.

An alternative to breastmilk that has been used successfully is a combination of the following: one third raw goat's milk, one third freshly extracted carrot and celery juice, and one third distilled water. The carrot and celery juice combination consists of about two–thirds carrot juice and one–third–celery juice. This will help overcome the folate deficiency of goat's milk. "...Goat's milk is actually more digestible, being richer in fats and having smaller protein molecules than cow's milk."[47]

It is important to secure goat's milk from a reliable source. Since it is illegal in most states to sell raw goat's milk, a person can buy partial interest in a goat and use the milk their goat is producing. Once there is no longer a need for the milk, the interest can be sold back to the former owner. Your local feed store owner may be able to help you locate someone who raises dairy goats.

It may also be helpful to consider adding about one half teaspoon of Udo's Choice Perfected Oil Blend to two or three feedings daily to help ensure adequate intake of the EFAs. As discussed earlier, DHA plays a vital role in the first year. Mothers will want to consider the benefits of supplementing with DHA if the infant is not being breastfed. Several companies market an excellent vegetable source of DHA developed by Martek and marketed under their brand names. Natrol, Nature's Way, Solaray, Source Natural's, Solgar, and Vitamin World are a few brands that are normally readily available. One gelcap punctured with the content added to one feeding daily should ensure that adequate DHA is supplied to the baby to support normal brain and retina development.

Since I have earlier pointed out the importance of B–12 in the diet, I should also mention that many parents may want to consider the benefit of crushing a sublingual B–12 supplement and adding a very small amount to the infant's diet two to three times each week *if the infant is not being breastfed*. One other area some mothers like to consider is the intestinal flora. As pointed out earlier, while breastfeeding, the infant is getting the benefit of the friendly flora associated with mother's milk. To ensure an infant has a well–balanced gastrointestinal flora, some mothers have found it beneficial to incorporate a probiotic supplement into one bottle daily.

Realizing it may be difficult for some parents to find fresh raw goat's milk, perhaps we should consider the possibility of resorting to pasteurized goat's milk. Ideally, it should be organic goat's milk from a local health food store. Since the naturally occurring enzymes have been destroyed in the pasteurization process, it may be helpful to obtain a good digestive enzyme supplement, open the capsule, and add to each serving. It is important to consider the naturally occurring components of mother's milk that may be missing from any substitute chosen, and then take the necessary steps to supply them. The same combination of fresh carrot and celery juice and distilled water as previously mentioned would be used.

While I'm sure there are many questions associated with the topic of breastfeeding and alternatives, it is important for us to realize that man cannot improve on God's provisions. I don't think there is any doubt that breastfeeding should be given the utmost consideration it deserves. The ultimate consideration should be for the long–term benefit and well–being of the newborn infant.

There are many good resources available that help teach couples the importance of breastfeeding and the best techniques to employ to make this a very successful and rewarding experience for everyone involved. I would encourage you to search them out and thoroughly educate yourself in this area. See the resource section of this booklet for some suggested sources.

Commercial formulas simply are not an ideal option. Although scientifically created to meet basic needs, they are nonetheless a "dead" processed food. Many are soy based, thus rich in the isoflavones and phytoestrogens.

> "Compared to babies who are fed soy or cow's milk–based formulas, babies who are breastfed for at least six months have three times fewer ear infections, five times fewer urinary tract infections, five times fewer serious illness of all kinds, seven times fewer allergies, and are fourteen times less likely to be hospitalized. . . . [F]or every 87 formula–fed babies who die from Sudden Infant Death Syndrome, only three breast–fed babies die from the disease. Babies who are fed only human milk for at least six months are six times less likely to develop lymphoma, a cause of cancer, in children."[48]

The evidence for the advantages of breastfeeding is overwhelming. Infants who are breastfed by vegetarian or vegan mothers have all these advantages plus much more, since their milk is far less contaminated with pesticides and other toxic chemicals.

Testimony: From Stephanie McGovern in Maryland: *"I am a 33-year-old mother of two daughters, ages 3½ and 18 months. My husband and I started the diet after becoming Health Ministers in the spring of 1996. I became pregnant six months later (no problems conceiving) and continued on the diet throughout my pregnancy and am still eating the Hallelujah way today.*

"Both of my pregnancies were wonderful. I had good health and energy. I was able to exercise regularly and keep up with a two-year-old at the park during my second pregnancy. I experienced no morning sickness. I gained 25 lbs. with both pregnancies.

"My girls were both beautifully healthy when they came into this world. Their complexions were clear and with good color. They were both very alert at birth. I did not use any drugs during labor.

My first daughter weighed 6 lbs. 15 oz. and my second daughter weighed 7 lbs. 3 oz.

"I nursed my first daughter until 20 months, at which time she weaned very naturally. My 18-month-old is still nursing, although only a couple of times a day. We have chosen not to vaccinate our girls and are very comfortable with our decision even though many people disagree with us.

"I began giving my girls dehydrated barley juice powder at six weeks of age—only 1/8 teaspoon in a little distilled water. They love it and now both take it twice a day. (3-year-old: 1 teaspoon twice a day, and 18-month-old: ½ teaspoon twice a day). They drink carrot juice once a day too. I give them B-12 twice a week, flax oil once a day, and in the winter months a supplement for vitamin D (we don't get out in the sun much in the winter).

"I introduced solids at about 9 months of age. I began with bananas, avocado, raw applesauce, raw sweet potato (in Champion juicer), and any other fruit that was soft. My first daughter began eating cooked food at about 16 months of age, very simple foods like brown rice and lentils, cooked veggies, potatoes, and almond butter on rice cakes. My 18-month-old is still eating mostly raw, she will occasionally eat a cooked veggie and she likes munching on rice cakes. Both girls drink almond milk that I make at home.

"We all enjoy good health. My 3-year-old has gotten a couple of colds each winter, but they are never very bad and they don't last long. She usually doesn't have much mucus; it's more congestion. She has had a couple of fevers that we just let run their course. My 18-month-old has been very healthy.

"Some of the biggest challenges to raising kids on this diet are making sure they always have something good to eat when we are visiting others or participating in group activities. When we visit my in-laws, I always bring a cooler full of food, plus two bags. Whenever we get together with other moms and their kids, I always have snacks on hand. Another challenge is spending a lot of time in the kitchen.

"Since my daughter was able to understand, I have always tried to explain to her our food choices. I let her know that we eat in a special way and that her friends eat another way. She knows what foods we eat and don't eat. It makes it easier to tell her "no" when she knows the reason. I always provide special treats when I know her other friends or cousin will be having something special.

"This Halloween I bought our 3-year-old some treats at our organic co-op (fruit leather, raisin packs, nut bars). When we took her trick-or-treating, my husband sneaked the good treats into her bag. When we got home, she was so excited to have some treats she could enjoy (without sugar), and the sugar candy, we put in a bag for her PopPop, who still eats the SAD diet. You just have to be creative with your kids."

C H A P T E R   5

Introducing Solid Foods

Train up a child in the way he should go: and when he is old,
he will not depart from it. —Proverbs 22:6

N ot only are parents responsible for the spiritual nurturing of their children, but also for instructing and showing them how to care for the body God has entrusted to them, to serve them throughout their life here on earth. When children learn early in life how to nourish their body in accord with God's natural laws, they can expect to enjoy optimal health here on planet earth until God calls His followers to their heavenly home.

Testimony: Dawn Lucie, from Florida, writes, *"I have two sons who are now 20 and 17. During both pregnancies, I ate probably 75% raw and drank lots of carrot juice. (Most people were utterly shocked that I never drank milk while pregnant or nursing.) During neither pregnancy did I ever experience morning sickness, swollen ankles, or have any complaint. Both deliveries were natural births with the assistance of a midwife. Both babies were exclusively on breast milk for a full year. During the second year, I added mashed banana and avocado to their breast milk diet. I did extensive research on the question of vaccinations, and as a result, my boys were NEVER inoculated! I think that because they never had dairy or meat products and were never vaccinated while growing up, they enjoyed wonderful health and never suffered such things as ear infections, colds, flu, etc. I feel good that I gave them a good start in life, and through the years have observed what marvelous health these boys have enjoyed."*

As we look at the introduction of the first solid foods, we need to once again keep in mind that there is much disagreement among the so-called "experts." It is important for the new parents to do their own research in this area and to be fully convinced in their own mind as to what is best for their baby. It is their responsibility to discern truth from error and to teach that truth to their children.

Keep in mind that babies born to vegetarian and vegan mothers may be a little slimmer than those of mothers on the SAD. Dr. Klaper notes that the average child in the United States is too fat! Sixty percent of all American children are obese (over 30% of their body weight is fat). We do not need to compare the birth weight and size of a healthy vegan baby to the same standards set for babies born to mothers on the SAD. Without a doubt, the vegan baby is the one who is "normal" according to God's timetable of development. The average, "normal" child today, as we said earlier, is too fat. They reach puberty years too early, from an average age of 16 years for girls during the 1940s to an average age of around 11 years today, with some girls finding the onset of menstruation even earlier than age 11.[49]

As noted by John Scharffenberg, M.D., M.P.H., medical nutritionist and Associate Professor of Applied Nutrition, Loma Linda University: "The average, so-called 'normal' child matures too rapidly here in the United States . . . It is known that vegetarian children mature later, begin menstruating later in life, have a delayed growth spurt, but do end up as tall as others, and their adult teeth emerge later in their childhood."[50] A diet that delays premature growth decreases cancer risk and cardiovascular disease in adulthood.

There is no hurry to introduce solid foods if the baby is content with nursing alone. Throughout the first eighteen to twenty-four months, the baby will continue to breastfeed as solid foods are introduced. Regardless of when weaning takes place, we must remember that there is never a time when cow's milk should be introduced into the diet. It is not and never will be an appropriate food for human consumption. There is an excellent book by Frank A. Oski, M.D., which addresses this whole issue. In regards to cow's milk, Dr. Oski has stated, "Milk has something for everybody. Who can argue with that? Of course that something might be diarrhea, iron-deficiency anemia, or even a heart attack."[51] Dr. Oski has an impressive record of service in pediatrics. In 1963, he was appointed as an Associate in the Department of Pediatrics at the University of Pennsylvania School of Medicine. In 1972 he assumed the position of Professor and Chairman, Department of Pediatrics, State University of New York, Upstate Medical Center. In 1985, he became Director, Department of Pediatrics, John Hopkins University School of Medicine and Physician–in–chief, the Johns Hopkins Children's Center.

Birth to Six Months

"Breastmilk is the perfect food for human babies and is all the vast majority of babies need until the middle of the first year of life (around 6 months)."[52] Babies are perfectly content to consume nothing but milk for several months. They generally are not ready for solid foods until they have doubled their birth weight, can hold their heads up, sit upright without help, and reach and grab for objects while sitting without assistance.[53] They will often begin grabbing for food when sitting on mother's lap if she is eating and try putting it into their mouths. Parents can exercise some simple common sense and observe natural signs that their baby is ready for solid foods. As they see the front teeth beginning to appear, they can be fairly certain the time for solid foods is approaching. It is also important to remember that breastmilk is the ideal and exclusive food for at least the infant's first six months. There is no need for adding water, juice, or any other supplement when the infant is exclusively breastfed. These could only confuse the infant.

As the baby grows older, changes are taking place with the whole digestive system. The stomach capacity is increasing and more milk can be consumed per feeding. The fat content of the milk is increasing, digestion takes a little longer, and more time may lapse between feedings. The body is producing more enzymes; and by the age of three months, the starch–splitting enzymes ptyalin and amalyse are close to levels found in adults. By the age of four months, the vision has matured and many things will divert the baby's attention from feeding. He will also be attracted to a greater variety of foods that he sees. By the age of six months, a baby's swallowing becomes voluntary, and he can hold food in his mouth, spit it out, or swallow it at will.

"One developmental sign of readiness for solid foods is the disappearance of the tongue extrusion reflex. The extrusion reflex allows infants to swallow only liquid foods. As long as this reflex persists, infants will push solids out of the mouth with their tongue, so that feeding such foods will be difficult."[54] Often developmental signs are better indicators of a child's readiness for certain foods than age guidelines. It is important to be flexible while adhering to general feeding guidelines.

Six Months to One Year

Around six months of age is a good time to begin introducing freshly extracted fruit juices diluted with about 50% distilled water. Fresh juices should be gradually introduced and may work up to a four-ounce serving within a week or two. The dilution with distilled water may gradually be reduced so that by twelve months the juice is consumed full strength unless the stools get too loose. After a few fruit juices have been introduced and are tolerated well, vegetable juices may be introduced. A favorite to begin with is carrot/celery juice diluted with distilled water. It is important to remember that infants who are exclusively breastfed should not need anything other than breastmilk for approximately the first six months. The exception to this is for infants who are not breastfed and who need the best substitute for breast milk as can be found.

We must remember that beginning solid foods is not an indication that weaning time is approaching. Nursing should continue for the first eighteen to twenty-four months or longer. We must also keep in mind that too early an introduction of solid foods decreases the child's desire to nurse and increases the chances of developing allergies.[55] There is ample evidence that the natural weaning age of a baby is not until sometime after the age of two. There are many long-term benefits associated with breastfeeding until at least the age of two or longer.

The Hunza people, some of the most extensively studied vegetarians in the world, have a reputation for being some of the healthiest and longest-living people in the world. Their children are breastfed until the age of three years. "Because the Hunza diet is an excellent one, good health is passed by the mother to the child, as described by G. T. Wrench in *The Wheel of Health*: '. . . the breast milk of the Hunza woman is as much derived from the Hunza food as is the blood of her womb.

Her breastfeeding is only a continuation of the period when she is an intervener between her offspring and the Hunza diet. The breast milk itself is a specially manufactured method of conveying that diet to the child."[56]

"By the age of six months, a baby can begin to eat solid foods. Swallowing becomes voluntary; a baby can hold food in the mouth, spit it out, or swallow it at will. Pancreatic fluid and other digestive juices are nearly like an adult's and are able to digest more complex proteins and carbohydrates."[57]

Now that it is time to begin adding some solid foods, where do you begin? Some believe when solid foods are introduced to a baby, they should be given one at a time; for example, give mashed bananas only on a particular day, and then observe how well they are tolerated before introducing a different fruit or other food. "Give the baby's digestive system a few days (up to a week) to get used to each new food before introducing additional ones."[58]

While Dr. Klaper feels it is best to introduce one food at a time, Dr. Jack Newman, whom we have referenced earlier, feels it is fine to introduce more than one food at a time. He indicates it is important to let the child experiment with various foods as he shows an interest in them. If there is an appropriate food (fruits initially) on your plate that he shows an interest in, mash it up and let him try it. His point is that we don't want to discourage his interest in solid foods. It would be a good idea to have the appropriate foods on mother's plate, as the baby is sitting in a high chair at the table during mealtime, to allow him to taste them and satisfy his curiosity as it develops.

It may be good to begin introducing solid food a few minutes after nursing just to let the baby get used to the texture and taste, beginning with ¼ teaspoon of mashed banana. We should remember we are not trying to fill him up, but simply introduce the new food to him. If he turns his head away or tightly closes his mouth, you can assume he is telling you he has had enough.

As he becomes more accustomed to the taste and texture he will begin demanding more. Keep in mind that a baby may not immediately like the taste of a specific food. Don't force it on him, but offer it to him on several different occasions. As his taste buds begin to mature he will grow accustomed to the taste and begin enjoying it after a few introductions.

This is an excellent time to help the infant to begin developing the good habit of thoroughly chewing (masticating) his food. Thoroughly masticating the food will help avoid digestive problems and nutritional imbalances later in life. Maximum absorption and utilization of the nutrients from our food is accomplished only when the fibers have been broken down by thorough mastication so the digestive juices can efficiently complete their breakdown of the food for assimilation.

After the baby is doing well with the mashed banana, avocado can be added and mashed with the banana. This offers an excellent source of good fats as well. "It is well not to introduce solid foods for five or six months (until front teeth appear), and then only mashed or strained raw fruits such as banana, avocado, scraped apple, pear, peach, apricot, sweet plum, etc. Cooked cereals introduced at a few weeks, or meat puree, puddings, and sugar sweetened cooked fruits will almost assuredly cause baby to be allergy–prone. . . . Infants lack the digestive enzymes for assimilation. These undigested foods become toxins, the beginning of problems for the tiny body."[59]

Fresh raw fruit is the ideal food to lead the transition while continuing with nursing. It is better to avoid the acidic fruits, such as oranges and grapefruits, until at least the baby's first birthday, and to exclude canned fruits altogether. Raw foods can be pureed in a number of ways. The Green Star or Champion juicers are ideal for this. During the next several months, a variety of fresh raw and cooked fruits can be added.

Testimony: Nicole Nixon writes, *"My children's diets are simple. My one–year–old drinks my breast milk for his main nourishment. I did not introduce anything else as a source of main nourishment until he had six teeth and he started demanding more food. He nurses in the morning and again at lunch. I knew his system was ready for some ripe fruits when he started consistently fussing for more to eat after the lunch nursing. Now at lunch, he gets one really ripe banana or half of a ripe, mushy pear cut into bite size pieces. He sets his own proportions. He stops eating when he is full. After lunch, he takes a nap and then nurses again right when he wakes up. Then he nurses before dinner, and I let him sit in his* *high chair with the family at the table while we eat dinner. He gets to chew on things that we have at the dinner table such as avocado slices, tomato pieces, lettuce leaves, cucumber slices, celery sticks, or broccoli bushels. If he can eat it and swallow it, that is fine with me. I have learned that he will not swallow anything his system is not ready for. He has a natural gag reflex that rejects anything that is not suitable for him at the stage he is at. He recently started to actually eat the tomatoes, but the other veggies just get gnawed into pieces and end up back on the high chair tray. He nurses one more time before going to bed for the night. He still wakes up for a middle of the night nursing. I always feed him when he is hungry. His little body is growing so fast right now, and he needs a lot of nourishment. I would not deprive him of that."*

The ideal time to begin adding raw pureed or blended vegetables to the child's diet will be when the molars begin to appear. When the digestive system is ready and able to handle more diverse foods, the teeth begin to appear to allow for eating these foods. Vegetable salads consisting of dark green leafy lettuce, a little fresh applesauce, carrot/celery juice, and a portion of an avocado can be blended in a blender or Vita–Mix to begin introducing raw vegetables into the diet. As more teeth erupt, less processing and pureeing will be required.

Mom and dad may want to have a blended salad at dinner to help peak the child's interest in them. There are many advantages to including blended salads in the diet. Unfortunately, many people eat their food in haste and neglect to masticate it thoroughly. Liquefying the vegetables in a blender is one way around this. Once blended, these foods are much easier to digest and the nutrients are more readily available for assimilation and utilization. We can also consume a greater volume of raw foods with less time spent on chewing and mastication. A variety of herbs may be added to enhance and vary the flavors for the adults who have not fully developed the taste for these delicious raw foods in a blended form. A young child should not need these as their taste buds have not been corrupted by the Standard American Diet.

Fresh steamed vegetables such as green beans, green peas, or carrots, as well as baked sweet potatoes or yams, may be mashed or pureed and introduced as well, after the molars begin to appear.

It is also important to take care of the baby's teeth as they are developing while nursing is continued. If the residue of sweets is left in the mouth, it can ferment and contribute to tooth decay. A small sip of purified water may be helpful immediately after nursing or eating fruit to rinse the sugars out of the mouth. It is also a good habit for adults to get into. Immediately after consuming a glass of carrot juice or eating a piece of fruit, it is a good idea to rinse the mouth with purified water.

During this process of introducing solid foods, it is important for the parents to relax and realize they can make this whole process a very rewarding experience. Their baby is being nourished with all of the vital nutrients required to promote optimal health through mother's milk or the selected alternative to mother's milk that is being provided. They can relax and enjoy the baby's exploration of various foods as he handles, smells, and taste them. Enjoy this time as he explores a new world of choices under your gentle guiding hand.

Right Time for the Right Food

As solid foods are being introduced, it is wise to be selective in food choices. Spinach and beets may contain excessive amounts of nitrates and should be avoided until at least ten to twelve months of age.

As the baby begins teething, many mothers introduce teething biscuits and crackers. It is important to avoid the highly processed white flour products. The toasted end slice of whole grain bread is a much better choice. It is vital to keep in mind that the baby must be supervised at all times when he is handling food. We do not want to allow an opportunity for him to choke on a piece of food.

Around ten months of age, starchy foods such as well–cooked baked potato (mashed with a little breast milk) and whole grain cooked cereals may be introduced. The more common organic whole grains such as brown rice, millet, barley, oats, and rye may be cooked and then run through a baby food grinder to make a paste, or the whole grains can be ground into a powder with a food mill and then cooked as needed. The grains may be blended with breast milk, raw goat's milk, nut milk, banana milk, or organic apple juice. Organic whole grains are a rich source of B vitamins, iron, and some trace elements.

Legumes (dried beans, peas, and lentils) should not be included until after twelve months of age. They are harder to digest than grains due to their enzyme inhibitors. Legumes should be soaked overnight and then slow–cooked until soft. The skins should be removed before they are ground or mashed to enhance digestibility. Legumes, like the grains, may also be ground into a powder and the powder may be cooked as needed. However, soybeans should be avoided. They contain larger amounts of digestive enzyme inhibitors, and larger amounts of the mineral binding phytic acid than any other legume. Along with being difficult to digest, they also inhibit the body's use of minerals.

Nuts and seeds can be used to produce some delicious milk and butters. Almonds are the best nuts as they leave an alkaline residue in the body. To make almond milk, soak the almonds overnight covered in purified water. In the morning drain the water, remove the skins, and blend a few almonds with enough purified water to produce a milk–like consistency (2 or 3 previously soaked, pitted dates may be added for sweetness). The milk may be strained and used as desired.

Nut and seed butters may be made in a masticating juicer by following the manufacturer's directions.

Some ideas for nut and seed milks:

Almond Milk

½ cup raw almonds
1 pint purified water
1 to 3 organic pitted dates or 1 tbs. maple syrup

Soak almonds 18 to 24 hours; drain water, remove the skins, rinse, and drain. Soak dates overnight in small container with just enough purified water to cover (dates with soaking water will be used). Blend all ingredients in a blender until smooth and creamy. Strain through a fine strainer or cheesecloth. Milk may be kept 24 to 48 hours in refrigerator.

Almond Sesame Milk

¼ cup raw almonds
¼ cup organic sesame seed
1 pint purified water
1 to 3 organic pitted dates or 1 tbs. maple syrup

Soak sesame seed 8 to 12 hours, drain, rinse and drain. Complete preparation as with almond milk.

Notes:

• Vegetable juices and/or avocado may be added to nut milks to make them more nutritious.
• One to two teaspoons of Red Star Nutritional Yeast may be added to nut milks as a good source of B–12.

Creamy Banana Milk
(from *Recipes for Life from God's Garden* by Rhonda Malkmus)

1 quart distilled water
½ ripe banana
½ to 1 cup sunflower seeds
3 tbs. raisins or 4 to 5 dates

Soak sunflower seeds overnight, and drain. Place all ingredients in blender and blend for 2 minutes. For thicker milk, add more banana.

Dr. N. W. Walker, in his book *The Vegetarian Guide to Diet & Salad,* offers the following recipe: "Put the following into the bowl of one of the little electric nut and seed grinders, which can be obtained from your health food store.

• 2 Tbs. raw shelled sunflower seeds
• 12 whole raw almonds with skin on
• 1 Tbs. whole sesame seeds

Grind to a very fine powder then put it in your blender with 1 pint of warm water and 1 tbs. of mild honey and thoroughly blend at high speed for 2 or 3 minutes. This is then ready to serve. . . ."[60]

Do not use honey for children under twelve months of age. Maple syrup may be substituted.

Generally by eighteen months of age, most babies are ready for the wide range of regular family foods, pureed if necessary. We want to strive for a high percentage of the baby's diet to be raw foods, but we do not want to deprive them of solid foods for breakfast, lunch, or dinner. While we may include some cooked foods at each meal, we will also want to be sure to include some raw foods as well. We want to always keep in mind that babies and children require a higher percentage of calories from good protein and fats than adults as they are growing and developing.

By the time all of the teeth have appeared, the child will be able to eat most of the same foods as the parents with some attention to the special needs of growing children, which we will briefly discuss in the next chapter.

As we conclude this chapter on getting off to the right start, please remember that the intent of this book is to simply lay a practical and solid nutritional foundation on which parents can continue to build as their knowledge and understanding increases. The bottom line in evaluating any nutritional ideas or concepts is to compare them with the natural laws established by God at the beginning of human history. Realizing we do not live in the ideal conditions that were enjoyed by Adam and Eve, or even those of the Old Testament patriarchs, we must keep in mind that God's laws and ideals established in the beginning have not been done away with.

When we look in nature at the animal kingdom, we see that, apart from man's intervention, they generally continue to thrive and enjoy optimal health. The foods eaten by each animal, whether their diet is plant-based or animal-based is eaten totally raw and as found in nature. They reproduce healthy offspring that mature into healthy specimens of their particular species, and apart from man's interference, they remain disease free.

As we consider the dietary and lifestyle needs of a pregnant woman and then those of the infant she gives birth to, we need to see how we can best duplicate the ideals as established by God in the beginning, or come as close to them as possible. Certainly, the scientific achievements of man can add nothing to God's original design. It should be apparent to any intelligent human being that the more man does to the foods supplied by nature, the less beneficial and potentially harmful they become. If our children and the next generation are going to enjoy optimal health, we must get back to and maintain a plant–based diet, free of as many processed foods as possible.

The first five years of an infant's life sets the stage for disease factors later in life. Parents should begin their research into nutrition well before an infant is conceived. There is a wide variety of opinions and information available on this subject. The Word of God should be the standard with which to measure all other information.

CHAPTER 6

Special Considerations for Children

As the young child is transitioning to more solid foods and less breast-milk, there are some areas that deserve special consideration.

Protein

It is important to ensure that there is an adequate amount of protein in the diet. It is well for us to remember that 5 % of the calories in breast milk, which is the ideal food for babies, is from protein. While all of our fruits and vegetables contain some protein, it is important to include liberal amounts of green vegetables, whole grains, legumes, and raw nuts and seeds (in the form of butters and milks) in the growing child's diet. They are in the growing process and require more protein than adults. Raw nut butters may be made in the Green Star or Champion juicer. Almonds are the best of the nuts, since they actually leave an alkaline ash when assimilated. Peanuts, which are not nuts but rather legumes, should not be used. Nut and seed butters can be made into a creamy spread by adding a little Udo's oil, flax seed oil, fruit juice, or water. This can then be spread on celery sticks or used as a vegetable dip.

Fat

Along with liberal amounts of protein, it is equally important to ensure there is an adequate amount of good fats in the child's diet. Fat is important in hormonal development, brain and retina development, bone growth, cell membrane integrity, and the assimilation of many of the vitamins and minerals. Sources of good fats are avocados, raw nuts and seeds (butters, milks, and creams), flax seed (should be ground fresh for each use), flax seed oil, and Udo's Choice Perfected Oil Blend. The oils may be added to blended salads, vegetables once the plate has been served (do not cook the vegetables with the oils), mashed with a baked potato, on a piece of whole grain toast, etc. They are very versatile and may be used in a variety of ways to ensure adequate intake of the essential fats. Walnuts are also an excellent source of the Omega 3 fats.

Vitamin B-12

As mentioned earlier, it is necessary to ensure there is a source of B-12 in the diet of the child after he is weaned. The diet of children who are not breastfed should also be supplemented with a small amount of vitamin B-12 as it is not readily available in our foods. Michael Donaldson, Ph.D., researcher for Hallelujah Acres Foundation, has found that one-half of a sublingual methycobalamin form of B-12 added to the child's diet twice a week should prevent the development of a B-12 deficiency.

Vitamin D

As presented in chapter two, vitamin D is actually a hormone manufactured by our body when sunlight falls upon the skin. It is essential for the absorption of calcium and phosphorus and is important for normal development of bones and teeth. With as little as an average of 15 minutes of sunlight daily, there should be no deficiency in this area. We must also remember that vitamin D made during the summer months can last through the winter, as it has been stored in the body by the liver. It is important to keep in mind that infants in northern climates with little exposure to sunshine may be in need of supplementation. Some research indicates that dark–skinned (especially African–American) babies may be in need of vitamin D supplementation since the darker–skinned individuals may need up to six times the exposure to sunlight to make adequate amounts of vitamin D. Your nutritionally minded health care provider should be consulted prior to vitamin D supplementation.

Some may wonder why we would need to consider supplementation with vitamin D if mother's breast milk is the ideal nutrition for an infant. As we mentioned, vitamin D is not a vitamin but rather a hormone manufactured by the body. Since it is not a nutrient, we would not expect it to be found in breast milk. The problem lies with the fact that our present day lifestyle and living conditions have adversely affected the production of this hormone in some instances due to our limited exposure to sunshine.

It may be important at this point to consider the negative impact that soft drinks have on the body's calcium reserves. Soft drinks contain high levels of phosphates that contribute to high levels of blood phosphates. When phosphates are high and calcium levels low in the blood, the body pulls calcium out of the bones. Thus soft drinks may be a major contributor to poor bone and teeth development in children, as well as osteoporosis in later years. There is no place in the diet for soft drinks for those desirous of optimal health. They should never be introduced to children.

Not only do the phosphates have a major negative impact on health, but also the massive amount of refined sugars impairs the immune system. The average 12–ounce soft drink contains approximately 10 to 12 teaspoons of sugar. "Research has shown that 24 teaspoons of sugar eaten in one day reduces the number of bacteria that our white blood cells will destroy by 92 percent."[61]

Child Development

"The first year of life is one of tremendous physical growth for which a high nutritive intake is essential. Babies under eight or nine months cannot tolerate an unhealthy diet. A good diet is so closely tied to normal development at this point in life that undernourishment usually shows up quickly."[62]

After the child is weaned and up to around three years of age, the child's eating patterns focus around those of the family. The parent has control over the child's diet. This is the time to begin reinforcing good eating habits.

It is common for the two–year–old to need help with feeding, and it may be difficult at times to prevent him from just playing with his food. They may have a decreased appetite, as the growth is slower than it was during the first two years.

From two to four years of age, table manners are being established. Many questions as to why, how, and what are being expressed as the child seeks to define his boundaries and take more control. Food preferences are becoming more important and are determined to a greater extent by taste.

Often by the age of five, food preferences have been established, and it is increasingly more difficult to find acceptance for new dishes and combinations. It is good to have developed a taste for a wide variety of foods by this age. As the child enters pre–school, peer pressure will begin to influence his desire for certain foods. It is important that a good foundation has been laid, so the child will continue to develop healthy eating patterns.

Once a child has entered school, social events, and settings will begin to influence eating patterns. If he has been well educated and trained up to this point, it will be easier for him to make the appropriate choices when faced with them. It is important to develop relationships with families who hold to similar nutritional standards in order to help direct the child in developing friendships that support his particular lifestyle. On-going education and support are crucial as many of the life–long dietary habits are being established.

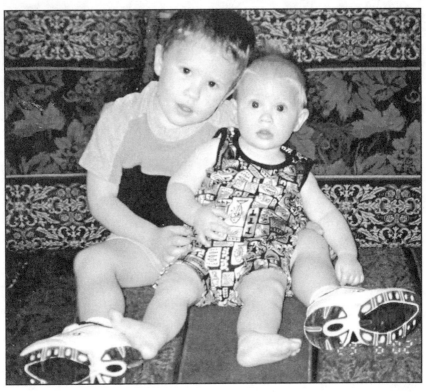

Dylan and Zachary Malkmus—You guessed it…Rev. Malkmus' grandchildren.
Their mother has been on The Hallelujah Diet® since long before pregnancy and the boys have been since birth.

C H A P T E R   7

Transitioning Children from the SAD to a Plant–based Diet

Testimony: Kathy Raine, from New York, writes: *"When I went on The Hallelujah Diet, I had my 2 children eating a lot of raw fruit and veggie snacks at first, but they still ate a lot of cooked food, too. As I was reading* Raw Kids *by Cheryl Stoycoff for ideas of how to move my children toward a more raw diet, it dawned on me that it can't be that hard, or even if it was, it would be more than worth it. My son is 6, and he needs a lot of help with a hot temper. My daughter is 11, and while she doesn't have any acute health problems, I truly believe this diet is the best you can do for your children.*

"I use all my creativity to make raw dishes to tempt them. Stoycoff has many good ideas in her book. My children have apple/carrot juice to start the day, then a big fruit salad with sprouted buckwheat, cinnamon, and raisins. If they get hungry before lunch, we have more fruit, maybe grapefruit or apples. I did find that the first two weeks they ate almost all the time, and then it evened out. The funny thing is, before the raw, my son could go all morning without eating. Now he's hungry, and he loves the fruit/sprout salad. We take a walk outside before lunch, and then we have a raw veggie lunch. I try to vary their veggies, if only the presentation. They eat a lot of sugar snap peas, baby carrots, and apples, but I keep trying to work things in to broaden

the repertoire. In lesser proportion, they eat some raw nuts, smoothies, manna/Essene bread, and some cooked grains. I make a dip out of almond butter and apple juice. I also make 'biscuits' out of sprouted spelt berries, dates (not a lot), and cinnamon run through the juicer, then dehydrated.

"It can be a challenge to get them to try new things, and I'll be glad when they develop a taste for avocados, vinegar, pure carrot juice, etc. The thing that helps me the most is my attitude. I am resolved and happy to help my children on their raw diet. I try not to think it's hard. I concentrate on the immense benefits. My daughter had had very bad eczema before we went off dairy a few years back, and the worst of it did resolve, but little spots would keep coming back. Now we never see it. My son has been making steady, slow improvement in his mental state, but I really noticed it about 2 weeks after the start of the diet, when at an unexpected party he had a chocolate cupcake and vanilla ice cream. Within half an hour, he was crying in a heap on the floor, and I realized he hadn't done this in the last 2 weeks—something he used to do all the time! Hallelujah!

"I also know that since I have had such dramatic health improvements with the diet, I am firm in my belief about raising my children in the diet. It's hard to believe I ever doubted raising my children vegetarian when they were born, and now we're on the raw diet. When I do have doubts creep in (and who doesn't), I just compare my children with how they were before. I also compare them with other people's 'SAD children.' My son is pretty skinny, but so is my friend's boy, who eats lots of pizza, cereal, meat, etc. We also don't get all the illnesses going around.

"I am lucky to be a home schooling mom, and you can be sure we are studying health and diet in our curriculum."

Unfortunately, many parents learn about the vital role that nutrition and a primarily raw plant–based diet play in overall health after their children are a few years old. While it is much easier and better to start off on a good, living–food nutritional program before conception, tremendous benefits can be realized by making positive dietary changes at any time in life. The younger the person is when these changes are made, the easier they are to make, in many respects.

It can seem like an overwhelming task to change a child's diet from the standard fast food, junk food diet to a healthy, living foods diet. Fortunately, the benefits can be nearly miraculous. Many parents have found that their ADD and ADHD diagnosed children become perfectly normal with no medication after going on a basically raw plant–based diet. As we realize the long–term impact of nutrition on the physical, emotional, and mental well being, it becomes vitally important that we educate our children and help facilitate the necessary changes in their diet and lifestyle.

Realizing that many children may not adopt a 75–85% raw plant–based diet, we must recognize that the simple inclusion of more fresh fruits and vegetables and the exclusion of most, if not all, animal products will produce outstanding long–term health benefits.

It is important that you recognize the social and psychological aspects of diet for children. You must approach this issue in a manner that will help them embrace the positive changes rather than rebel against them. You must start from whatever point you are at and realize it is not too late to have a very significant positive impact on the health of your children.

Testimony: Nicole Nixon, from Texas, shares some personal insights in "A Word For Mothers With Picky Eaters": *"My 3–½ year-old is a 'veggie–boy' too. He was born and lived his first two years of life on the Standard American Diet. Switching him to The Hallelujah Diet was a long, slow, tedious process. Don't tell me your child is too picky of an eater for you to ever successfully change his diet. My 3–½ year old is king of picky eaters.*

"Here's what I did. I got a sheet of paper and wrote this Proverb in red ink: "He who is full loathes honey, but to the hungry even what is bitter tastes sweet. —Proverbs 27:7" and taped it to the refrigerator right at eye level. I decided I would ultimately win all food battles, but to keep the battles as un–traumatic as possible, first using positive reinforcement, but relying on negative reinforcement only as a last resort. Then, I made a cup of fresh apple juice with a tiny bit of carrot juice in it. I tasted it to make

sure it tasted good and sweet. Humans generally like sweet tasting things. I gave it to him and said, "Here's your apple juice." He tasted it and didn't like it. Not the same as the frozen concentrate stuff I had always given him before. He's a mule when it comes to change. Then I relied on a little college psychology, Pavlov's theory. If a dog receives an immediate, positive response or reward for a specific action, the dog will repeat the action or behavior in order to get the reward again. Eventually, you can remove the reward, and the dog will still perform the action. I figured if you could train a dog this way you can certainly train a child. The one healthy treat I could think of that my child really got excited about was raisins. So I said, 'Zane, do you want a raisin?' And he of course excitedly said yes. 'Okay, then take one drink of your juice and I will give you one raisin.' Finally, he decided that one drink would be worth one raisin. So we drank our juice, getting one raisin after every drink until the juice was gone. This worked most days. He did not get anything else until his juice was all gone. On some days, he would go well past lunchtime with nothing to eat, because he still had not finished his juice. He would eventually finish it, and then I would feed him other things.

"On really stubborn days, I would have to rely on negative reinforcers if the positive reward system wasn't working. It was so important to me that my child learned to drink fresh juice. 'Zane,' I would say, 'take a drink and get a raisin. If you do not take a drink you will be disobeying Mommy's instructions and what happens when we disobey?' And he would answer, 'Get a spanking.' I don't think I ever had to actually spank him for not drinking his juice. But if he had chosen to get a spanking rather than drinking his juice, I would certainly have given him one. It was his choice. And then he would still have to drink his juice. But like I said, it was only on the extremely stubborn days that I would even have to threaten a spanking. He ultimately would decide that taking a drink and getting a raisin was better than getting a spanking.

"The amount of carrot juice in the apple juice was very slowly increased over a gradual amount of time. Kind of like the frog that won't jump out of a pot of boiling water when he is placed *there while the water is still cool. Gradually, the water is heated to boiling and the frog never jumps because he cannot feel the heat when it is increased so gradually. The proportions now are 4 regular carrots to half an apple (or 2/3 carrot juice to 1/3 apple juice). Basically, it's carrot juice with a little apple juice in it. He had to drink each cup of juice using the reward system for a very long time. Eventually, he got used to the juice. I would give it to him with no word of rewards and use the rewards only when he would ask for them. Now he just drinks his juice. It's a habit, a ritual; he expects it every morning upon rising and every afternoon when he wakes up from his nap. He gets juice twice a day at these times, no questions asked. And he drinks it before he can have anything else. The day he ASKED for his juice was a glorious day. I was telling everybody, 'He asked for his juice this morning, can you believe it? My child actually asked for his carrot juice!'*

"Another trick was that I could not call it carrot juice. That just threw him into a mental disgust and he could not fathom tasting it. So I renamed it. Zane has been drinking 'Zane Juice' from the beginning . . . It was designed especially for his body to make him big, and strong, and smart. I bought a dark blue sippy cup especially for his 'Zane Juice' so that he could not see the color of the juice that disgusted him and created mental blocks as well. I made sure to strain the juice really well, because the pulp was another disgust factor. The final step was to slowly add dehydrated barley juice powder to his carrot juice. I started small (1/8 tsp.) and worked up to 1 tsp. of dehydrated barley juice powder in each cup of carrot juice. So that was the juice battle. You can ultimately win, but it takes patience, creativity, and knowing what will motivate your child."

Your Level of Competence

If you are going to be successful in transitioning your child to a healthy living foods diet, you will have to be confident and armed with the nutritional information your child needs to help him understand the importance of diet and lifestyle (if he is old enough to understand). Often older children feel they are in the peak of health and are invincible. Unfortunately, even young children are now battling chronic conditions such as cancer, diabetes, and heart disease. No longer are the young exempt from these life–threatening conditions. Since the advent of the fast food diet and lifestyle, the incidence of these diet–related diseases has increased significantly.

You must set the example. It doesn't work to tell your child one thing and then let him see you do something differently. If you haven't completely embraced the changes you are asking him to make, you can't expect him to readily follow along. You must set and adhere to the standard. You must be prepared for opposition from family and friends. Granddad or Grandma probably will not understand why you refuse to let you child 'enjoy' candy, bubblegum, and soft drinks when all the other kids are having those things. It isn't easy for you or your child to withstand peer pressure.

> **Testimony:** Tina Fillmer, from North Carolina, tells how she deals with grandparents: *"A recent problem I have found a solution for is the girls' sleepover with their grandparents. At one point, my mother would serve them 4 different treats in a row . . . 2 cookies, an ice cream bar, and a piece of hard candy. As soon as I found out about the healthy treat recipes, I made a deal with my Mom. I allowed one 'unhealthy' treat (it's difficult to expect my little 3 and 4–year–olds to not eat what my parents are eating) and I allow one 'healthy' treat. This seems to be working. Eventually, I will transition my Mother to only give them a 'healthy' treat."*

Continually reinforcing your beliefs through ongoing education is important. A good solid fundamental home study course, videos, audios, and books can prove to be of immeasurable value.

> Tina Fillmer has found education a key to her success: *"Another key theme with children is to EDUCATE them. My girls, although at young ages, understand why we don't drink cow's milk. Sometimes I serve them Rice Dream ice cream/ice cream bars and they ask me 'Mommy, does this have cow's milk in it?' When weaning them off cow's milk, I simply mixed part rice milk with the cow's milk and gradually added more and more of the rice milk and less cow's milk until they were drinking 100% rice milk.*

They never complained or even noticed. (They do not drink rice milk everyday.)"

Enlisting Your Child's Help

If your child is old enough, you should carry on an honest conversation with him or her as to why you want to change his or her diet. If there is some immediate benefit that he can expect, he will be more inclined to embrace the changes. If he has any learning difficulties in school, you could point out the impact diet has in this area. If he is athletic, you could mention to him some of the vegetarian athletes who have excelled in sports, such as, Dave Scott, the six time winner of the Iron-man Triathlon; Bill Pearl, four time Mr. Universe; Martina Navratilova, tennis champion; Andreas Cahling, champion body–builder and gold medal winner in the ski jump; Hank Aaron, all time great major league baseball player. (See page 136 in *God's Way to Ultimate Health* by Rev. George Malkmus for other vegetarian athletes.)

> Tina Fillmer has found: *"An EXCELLENT time to educate them 'gently' is when they're sick. They know that healthy people eat lots of fruits and vegetables and people who are sick probably do not. My 4–year–old, after being sick with a cold for a week, suddenly became much more interested in drinking her carrot juice and dehydrated barley juice powder. I explained to her that these foods help prevent us from getting sick. There was a change in her attitude. I guess she realized that she could avoid getting sick and just didn't want to feel lousy again. Today, she surprised me when she informed me that she runs much faster than my 3–year–old because she eats tomatoes and her little sister doesn't. She understands cause and effect better than most adults I know . . . when it comes to health."*

Just realizing how simple the diet and lifestyle can be will appeal to many children. Having a fruit smoothie one morning and a bowl of whole grain cereal the next morning can be more like a special treat than a meal. (A great raw cereal can be made by mixing organic rolled oats, almonds [slivered or ground], and freshly ground flax seed, and adding organic apple juice or homemade almond milk.) This may be eaten as a cold raw cereal. Also, you may heat one cup of the apple juice, remove from heat, add ½ cup of the mixture, cover and let stand 15 to

20 minutes for a warm cereal. This or a comparable cereal could be prepared and sent with a child to school in a thermos bottle.

Lunch at home with mother for the preschooler could be a blended salad followed by a bowl of garden vegetable soup (or any variety of homemade soups). Dinner may begin with a salad (blended for those younger children who don't chew the vegetables thoroughly), followed by some baked or steamed vegetables, whole grains, legumes, or a whole grain pasta with homemade tomato sauce. A serving of fresh vegetable juice can be worked in mid–morning and mid–afternoon, or thirty minutes before the meal. Fruit (fresh and dried), as well as raw nuts and seeds, should be available for between–meal snacks. At least a couple of servings of a properly processed concentrated green juice (low temperature dried barley juice, not a whole leaf product) should be worked in daily, as well. Secure some of the recipe books listed in the resource section for more ideas.

For the school age child, lunch can offer special opportunities. It is important for him to first of all understand why he eats the way he does. He should understand that he has knowledge about the correct way to nourish his body that few children have. This should not be a concept of superiority but rather a feeling of peace and assurance that he will not have to experience the physical problems most of his peers will experience. This can be a tremendous opportunity for him to be a witness and testimony to those he associates with on a daily basis.

> **Testimony:** For those with a "picky eater," Nicole offers further insights from her experience in transitioning her son Zane to a plant–based diet: *"The rest of his diet was a battle, too, but not so much as the juice. This is where I relied heavily on Proverbs 27:7 that was posted on my refrigerator. There were a few healthy things I knew he liked and in the beginning that was pretty much all he ate. He liked apples dipped in raw honey (kids love to dip things), cantaloupe, and bananas. He liked oatmeal made with fresh apple juice (instead of milk), a little honey, and sprinkled with raisins. And he liked tomatoes and frozen peas (yes, straight out of the bag, frozen and all). He liked mashed potatoes and pasta of any kind. So that is what he ate. The killer foods were no longer an option, and if he didn't want what I fixed he could*

choose to not eat (Proverbs 27:7). And he knew I was serious. There was one time that he chose to not eat. When bedtime came and his little tummy was hungry, he got to go to bed hungry. It was very hard for me and my husband to put our child to bed hungry, but all it took was one time. He still slept that night. And when he woke up in the morning, he was ready to eat. He has never chosen to not eat since that time. I try to balance giving him the things I know he likes while encouraging him to try new things that I think he should like. As I said, I knew of the healthy things he would eat, and I made those staples of his diet. Every now and then I would encourage him to try something new. He would get a special day at the store to pick anything he wanted to try out of the fresh produce section. I would buy it for him to take home and try. Having these special shopping trips helped him to overcome his dislike of trying new things. He learned to love plums, cherries, mangos, pears, and some other fruits this way . . . Be firm, be in control, and don't let your child win the battles, but try to creatively make eating healthy stuff a positive experience."

For lunch, the child may take any variety of raw fruits, organic dried fruits, raw nuts and seeds, fresh vegetable sandwiches on whole grain bread, or a variety of warm soups or whole grain cereals in a thermos. On the days when the school offers reasonable choices in vegetables or vegetarian entrees, he or she may choose to eat in the cafeteria. Although usually not the best in quality, many schools offer a salad bar as an option. You may be able to take an active role in helping your school develop a more healthy lunch program.

The age of the children involved will be a major factor in the whole process of transitioning to a health dietary lifestyle. Young children under two years of age are relatively easy to transition over to healthy eating. The parents of home–schooled children will often find it relatively easy to keep their children on track. Many older teens will readily accept the whole concept of transitioning to a healthy diet and lifestyle. Others who feel they are almost grown up and eat out often may be reluctant to make the changes. It may be better not to try to force them to embrace the concept of a primarily raw diet, but to gently encourage them to make moderate changes that will offer life–long benefits. Each meal at home can begin with a fresh raw salad, followed with a good variety of fresh and baked vegetables they enjoy. Some of the more healthy meat and cheese substitutes may be worked into the diet in a way that they will be readily accepted.

It is important to remember that much of a person's core belief system has been established by the age of four. This is one reason that developing good dietary habits early in childhood is vital. Those habits will go with them throughout life unless there are some strong outside factors later in life that re-educate them and involve them emotionally with change. Likewise, it takes positive emotional involvement and education to overcome poor dietary habits that have been established since early childhood. We must work consistently, diligently, and patiently in helping the older child redefine the core belief system that was established in those earlier years of poor eating habits. Many of us as adults can recall the struggles we had as we worked at overcoming that core belief system when we first learned of the importance of a primarily raw plant-based diet. Not only did we have to reprogram our thinking, but we also had to deal with the negative pressures from well-meaning friends and family who thought we had totally "lost it" when it came to eating and lifestyle. They not only do not want to hear about our newfound diet and lifestyle, but they want to help us "get back on track" with the SAD.

Fortunately, when children are raised on The Hallelujah Diet® and their core belief system is established on a solid foundation in early childhood, they seldom yield to the temptations of unhealthy food choices.

> **Testimony:** Susan Matchett, from Ontario, Canada: *"In April 1996, we were loaned a video,* How to Eliminate Sickness. *We were so impressed with this video that we began following The Hallelujah Diet. Our daughter, Charlyne Kiah Matchett, was born on January 27, 1996. We three began enjoying the benefits of this diet.*
>
> *"When we planned our second child we continued following The Hallelujah Diet strictly. During the nine months of pregnancy, I enjoyed great health with no morning sickness. After a wonderful delivery, we were given a fine son, Riley Caleb Ferguet Matchett, born December 29, 1997.*

"Both Charlyne and Riley were breastfed four months. Their care is a pleasure! . . . In 1998, we added Rhonda's Recipes for Life from God's Garden to our library. This is a wonderful book from which we receive much guidance.

"The amazing thing about our children is that they will not eat junk foods or meats in any form even when other people offer it to them. We are pleased with their robust health and quick minds. Our introduction to the Hallelujah lifestyle has been most healthful and educational."

CONCLUSION

Almost daily over the past several years, I've been asked various questions about raising healthy children on a primarily raw plant–based diet. As a result of some of these questions, I found it necessary to do research to clarify some issues in my own mind first. Much of what is contained in this book is a result of that research and study. I trust it has helped in laying a sound basic nutritional foundation from which each parent can build as he or she takes charge of not only their own health, but also that of their children.

I learned some time back that information is always changing and that the area of nutrition is very controversial. I have found that as I encounter controversial issues, it is always helpful to first of all see if the Bible, the Word of God, addresses those issues. Almost always, I can find some basic guidelines from God's Word as I discover His natural laws that were established from the foundation of the world. We can rest assured that God's natural laws are unchanging, and that if what we do lines up with them, the outcome will be positive.

I appreciate the testimonies that many have shared with me as to their experiences in adopting The Hallelujah Diet® and in rearing healthy children on a primarily raw plant–based diet. Often it is much easier to learn from the personal experiences of others than it is to learn from documented research. I trust their testimonies have been a reinforcement of the basic message of health.

We learn from the parable of the sower and the seed in Matthew chapter 13 that not only do we reap what we sow, we reap more than we sow. The farmer plants a seed of corn and harvests hundreds of kernels from the ears this one seed produces.

We also learn from Hosea 8:7 that when we sow to the wind, we reap the whirlwind. While in the context these have spiritual applications, they also apply physically. What we sow in regards to nourishing the body is multiplied back to us. When we sow wisely, we reap optimal health. When we sow foolishly or to the wind, we reap impaired health, disease, and sickness.

I encourage you to invest some time in research and study so that you can make wise decisions in regards to your own health, as well as that of the children God entrusts to you. Rearing our children with sound, fundamental principles of physical health and well–being provides them with one of the greatest resources for living life to the fullest. Yet it is by far more important that we teach them how to enjoy a personal relationship with God through His Son, Jesus Christ, and to know without a doubt that after this temporal life here on earth is over that they will spend eternal life in heaven. The Bible teaches that it is very simple to know that we have assurance of eternal life in heaven.

Since Adam and Eve's original sin, we are born with physical life, yet spiritual death, with no capacity for fellowship with God in time or eternity. We are born under the penalty of sin, which is spiritual death and ultimate separation from God throughout eternity unless we personally accept Jesus Christ as our savior. (Romans 3:23, 6:23; Acts 4:12)

> For God so loved the world, that he gave his only begotten Son, that whosoever believeth in him should not perish, but have everlasting life. For God sent not his Son into the world to condemn the world; but that the world through him might be saved. —John 3:16–17

> That if thou shalt confess with thy mouth the Lord Jesus, and shalt believe in thine heart that God hath raised him from the dead, thou shalt be saved. For with the heart man believeth unto righteousness; and with the mouth confession is made unto salvation. —Romans 10:9–10

When your child is old enough to understand the gospel message, you can have the joy of leading him in understanding that Jesus Christ came to earth, lived a sinless life, was crucified on the cross, and rose from the dead to provide salvation for all who will accept His free gift. He bore the punishment for our sins on the cross as our substitute. He removed the sin barrier that separates us from God. We can simply go to God in prayer and acknowledge that we are sinners. We tell Him that we believe the Biblical record of the death, burial, and resurrection of Jesus Christ, and that we accept Him as our personal savior.

If you or your loved ones have never personally accepted God's gift of eternal life, I encourage you to do so today. Read the Gospel of John and the books of Romans and I John as you begin a new life in Christ. Not only does God want us to enjoy optimal health, but He also wants us to have daily fellowship with Him and ultimately to spend eternity with Him.

Beloved, I wish above all things that thou mayest prosper and be in health, even as thy soul prospereth. —3 John 2

If you or your child have accepted Jesus Christ as your savior and would like additional information, write to Hallelujah Acres requesting more literature in regards to salvation and the Christian life.

APPENDIX 1

Hallelujah Acres Resources
(704) 481–1700
www.hacres.com

Children and The Hallelujah Diet, Joel Robbins, M.D. (audio)

Diet for a New America and *Diet for a New World,* John Robbins

Don't Drink Your Milk, Frank A. Oski, M.D.

Fats that Heal, Fats that Kill, Udo Erasmus, Ph.D.

Feeding Our Children (video)

God's Way to Ultimate Health, Rev. George Malkmus with Michael Dye

Hallelujah Acres Home Study Course: Hallelujah Acres School of Natural Health, phone (704) 481–1700 or e-mail to school@hacres.com

Hallelujah Acres University

How to Eliminate Sickness, Rev. George Malkmus (audio and video available)

Miraculous Self-Healing Body Video

Recipes for Life . . . from God's Garden, Rhonda Malkmus

Reclaiming Our Health, John Robbins

Vaccinations: Deception & Tragedy, Michael Dye

APPENDIX 2
Other Resources

Information

"Alive," *Canadian Journal of Health and Nutrition* (periodical), 7436 Fraser Park Dr., Burnaby, BC, V5J JB9 Canada, phone (604) 435-1919, www.alivemagazine.com

"Alternative Medicine" (periodical), 1650 Tiburon Blvd., Tiburon, CA 94920, phone (415) 435-1779, www.alternativemedicine.com

La Leche League, P.O. Box 4079, Schaumburg, IL 60168-4079; phone (847) 519-7730 or (800) LA LECHE, <http://www.lalecheleague.org>. This organization helps women to be successful at breastfeeding.

Norman Clinical Laboratory, Inc. Cincinnati, OH, phone (800) 397-7408, www.b12.com.

"Vegetarian Times" (periodical), P.O. Box 570, Oak Park, IL 60303, www.vegetariantimes.com.

Supplements

Plant-based DHA supplements from Martek Bioscience are available under such brand names as Nature's Way, Solaray, Natrol, Source Naturals, Solgar, Pruitan's Prided, or Martek direct by calling 888-OK-BRAIN. www.martekbio.com

The following supplements are available from Hallelujah Acres by calling 800-915-9355 or by visiting the web site at www.hacres.com

BarleyMax®
B-Flax-D
Hallelujah Acres B-12, B-6 & Folic Acid
Barlean's Flaxseed Oil
Udo's Choice Perfected Oil Blend
Hallelujah Acres Children's Probiotic
Organic Golden Flaxseed

BIBLIOGRAPHY

The New Analytical Bible and Dictionary of the Bible, Authorized King James Version. Chicago: John A Dickson Publishing Co., 1973.

Anderson, James W. et al. "Breast–feeding and Cognitive Development: A Meta–Analysis." *The American Journal of Clinical Nutrition* 70(4) (1999): 525–35.

Erasmus, Udo. *Fats that Heal Fats that Kill.* Burnaby, British Columbia: Alive Books, 1986.

"Essential Supplements for the New Millennium." *Healthy and Natural Journal* (October 1998): reprint.

Finnegan, John. *The Facts About Fats.* Malibu, CA: Celestial Arts, 1993.

Holford, Patrick. *The Optimal Nutrition Bible.* Freedom, CA: The Crossing Press, 1997.

Jensen, Bernard. *Foods That Heal.* Garden City Park, NY: Avery Publishing Group, Inc., 1988.

Klaper, Michael. *Pregnancy, Children, and the Vegan Diet.* Maui, HI: Gentle World, Inc., 1987.

Malkmus, George H. *God's Way to Ultimate Health.* Shelby, NC: Hallelujah Acres Publishing, 1995.

Malkmus, Rhonda J. *Recipes For Life . . . from God's Garden.* Shelby, NC: Hallelujah Acres Publishing, 2001.

McDougall, John. *The McDougall Newsletter* (vol) (March/April 1997): 1–2.

Messina, Mark, and Virginia Messina. *Dietitian's Guide to Vegetarian Diets.* Gaithersburg, MD: Aspen Publishers, Inc., 1996.

Messina, Mark and Virginia Messina. *Total Health for You and Your Family.* New York: Virginia Three Rivers Press, 1996.

Messina, V.K. and K. L. Burke. *The Journal of the American Dietetic Association* 97: 1317–21.

Newman, Jack. *The Ultimate Breastfeeding Book of Answers.* Roseville, CA: Prima Publishing, 2000.

Oski, Frank A. *Don't Drink Your Milk.* Brushton, NY: Teach Services, Inc., 1983.

Oski, Frank A. "What We Eat May Determine Who We Can Be." *Nutrition* 13 (November 3, 1997): 220–221

Robbins, John. *Diet For A New America.* Tiburon, CA: H.J. Kramer Inc., 1998.

Robbins, John. *Reclaiming Our Health.* Tiburon, CA: H.J. Kramer Inc., 1996.

Swope, Mary Ruth. *Surviving The 20ᵗʰ Century Diet.* Phoenix, AZ: Swope Enterprises, 1996.

Walker, N.W. *The Vegetarian Guide to Diet & Salad.* Prescott, AZ: Norwalk Press, 1971.

Whitney, Eleanor Noss and Sharon Rady Rolfes. *Understanding Nutrition,* 8th ed. Belmont, CA: Wadsworth Publishing Company, 1999.

Yntema, Sharon. *Vegetarian Baby.* Ithaca, NY: McBooks Press, 1980.

Yntema, Sharon. *Vegetarian Children.* Ithaca, NY: McBooks Press, 1987.

NOTES

[1]Robbins, John, *Diet For A New America* (Tiburon: H J Kramer, Inc., 1998), 330.

[2]Whitney, Eleanor Noss and Sharon Rady Rolfes, *Understanding Nutrition,* eighth edition (Belmont: Wadsworth Publishing Company, 1999), 342–43.

[3]*The New Analytical Bible and Dictionary of the Bible* (Chicago: John A. Dickson Publishing Company, 1973), 90.

[4]Klaper, Michael, *Pregnancy, Children, and the Vegan Diet* (Maui: Gentle World, Inc., 1997).

[5]V. K. Messina and K. L. Burke, "Position of the American Dietetic Association: Vegetarian Diets," *J Am Diet Assoc* 11 (November 1997): 1317–1321; quoted in Whitney, *Understanding Nutrition,* 187.

[6]Physicians Committee for Responsible Medicine, "Vegetarian Diets: Advantages for Children," available from <http://www.pcrm.org/health/Info_on_Veg_Diets/vegetarian_kids. html>.

[7]McDougall, John, *The McDougall Newsletter,* available from <http://www.drmcdougall.com/march_april97.html>.

[8]Ibid.

[9]Messina, Virginia and Mark Messina, *The Vegetarian Way: Total Health for You and Your Family* (New York: Three Rivers Press, 1996), 159.

[10]Klaper, *Pregnancy, Children, and the Vegan Diet,* 1.

[11]Ibid., 2.

[12]The masculine pronoun is herein used in the generic sense to include either male or female.

[13]Firman E. Bear et al. 1948.

[14]Holford, Patrick, *The Optimum Nutrition Bible* (Freedom: The Crossing Press, 1999), 66–67.

[15]Jensen, Bernard, *Foods That Heal* (Garden City Park: Avery Publishing Group, Inc., 1993), 104.

[16]"Sanoviv Dietary Program," available from www.sanoviv.com/nutritiontext.htm.

[17]Whitney, *Understanding Nutrition,* 131.

[18]"Essential Supplements for the New Millennium," Healthy and Natural Journal (October 1998).

[19]Oski, Fran A., "What We Eat May Determine Who We Can Be," *Nutrition* 13 (Nov. 3, 1997): 220–21 (special reprint).

[20]Anderson, James W. et al., "Breast–feeding and cognitive development: a meta–analysis," *American Journal of Clinical Nutrition* 70(4) (1999): 525–35.

[21]Erasmus, Udo, *Fats that Heal, Fats that Kill* (Burnaby, BC: Alive Books, 1993), 7.

[22]Michael Donaldson, "Vitamin B–12 and the Hallelujah Diet," available from www.hacres.com/articles.asp?artid=105.

[23]Whitney, *Understanding Nutrition,* 480.

[24]Messina, *The Vegetarian Way,* 118.

[25]Klaper, *Pregnancy, Children,* 22.

[26]Whitney, *Understanding Nutrition,* 309–310.

[27]Ibid., 478.

[28]Messina, *The Vegetarian Way,* 163.

[29]Klaper, *Pregnancy, Children,* 17.

[30]Yntema, Sharon, *Vegetarian Baby* (Ithaca: McBooks Press, 1991),53.

[31]Robbins, John, *Reclaiming Our Health* (Tiburon: H J Kramer, 1996), 31.

[32]Ibid., 17.

[33]Ibid,. 19.

[34]Ibid., 19.

[35]Ibid., 25.

[36]Ibid., 27.

[37]Ibid., 25.

[38]*Journal of Asthma* 37 (2000): 589–94.

[39]Klaper, *Pregnancy, Children,* 32.

[40]"70 Percent of All Antibiotics Given to Healthy Livestock," Union of Concerned Scientists News, January 8, 2001, available from www.ucsusa.org/releases/01-08-01.html.

[41]Caughlan, Stacelynn, "Breastmilk Liquid Gold," *Alive Magazine,* September 2001, 28.

[42]Finnegan, John, "The Vital Role of Essential Fatty Acids For Pregnant and Nursing Women," available from www.thorne.com/townsend/dec/efas.html.

[43]Newman, Jack and Pitman, Teresa, *The Ultimate Breastfeeding Book of Answers* (Roseville: Prima Publishing, 2000), 46.

[44]Whitney, *Understanding Nutrition,* 505.

[45]Ibid., 505–6.

[46]Newman, *The Ultimate Breastfeeding Book,* 8.

[47]Yntema, *Vegetarian Baby,* 141.

[48]Robbins, John, "What About Soy?", available from www.foodrevolution.org/what_about_soy.htm.

[49]Klaper, *Pregnancy, Children,* 36–37.

[50]Ibid., 37.

[51]Oski, Frank, *Don't Drink Your Milk!* (Brushton: Teach Services, Inc., 1996), 67.

[52]Newman, *The Ultimate Breastfeeding Book,* 357.

[53]Messina, *The Vegetarian Way,* 176.

[54]Messina, Mark and Messina, Virginia, *the Dietitian's Guide To Vegetarian Diets* (Gaithersburg: Aspen Publishers, Inc. 1996), 263.

[55]Klaper, *Pregnancy, Children,* 34, 49.

[56]Yntema, *Vegetarian Baby,* 21–22

[57]Ibid., 111.

[58]Klaper, *Pregnancy, Children,* 49.

[59]Malkmus, Rhonda, *Recipes for Life from God's Garden* (Shelby: Hallelujah Acres Publishing, 2001), 99–100.

[60]Walker, N. W., *The Vegetarian Guide to Diet & Salad* (Prescott: Norwalk Press, 1995), 12.

[61]Swope, Mary Ruth, *Surviving The 20th Century Diet* (Phoenix: Swope Enterprises, 1996), 24.

[62]Yntema, Sharon, *Vegetarian Children* (Ithaca: McBooks Press, 1995), 20.